All You Have to Do Is Walk

Bliss on the Appalachian Trail

John Sievel, aka Will See

Dedication

This book is dedicated to all those who plan, build, maintain, conserve and support the Appalachian Trail. Their efforts made my journey possible.

Table of Contents

Why?

Bliss. That's what we feel. Bliss. Why? Where does it come from? That is what this book is about.

In 2012, I spent 4 1/2 months hiking almost 1000 miles of the A.T. (Appalachian Trail). The intensity blew me away. The trail infected me. I feel it almost every day. It changed me.

The book is organized in sections that reflect the geography of the trail, starting at Springer Mountain, GA, in the south, and ending in Maryland in the north. So it is helpful to read them in order, since that is the way the trail revealed itself to me. The connectivity and flow are important.

Most sections begin with a journal entry, that looks like this. The journal entries are lightly edited, and maintain much of the flavor that the trail imparted at the time.

After the journal entries, there usually is a section that looks like this. It contains my thoughts and memories of that particular time on the trial.

The following page is an index into detailed maps that show locations mentioned in the journal entries. The maps are not to scale, and should not be relied upon for actual hiking.

To long distance hikers, I owe an apology for my feeble, ineffective attempt to convey what we all feel inside.

To those who have never experienced a significant amount of time on a long distance hike, come walk with me and laugh, cry, hurt, and rejoice.

Maps

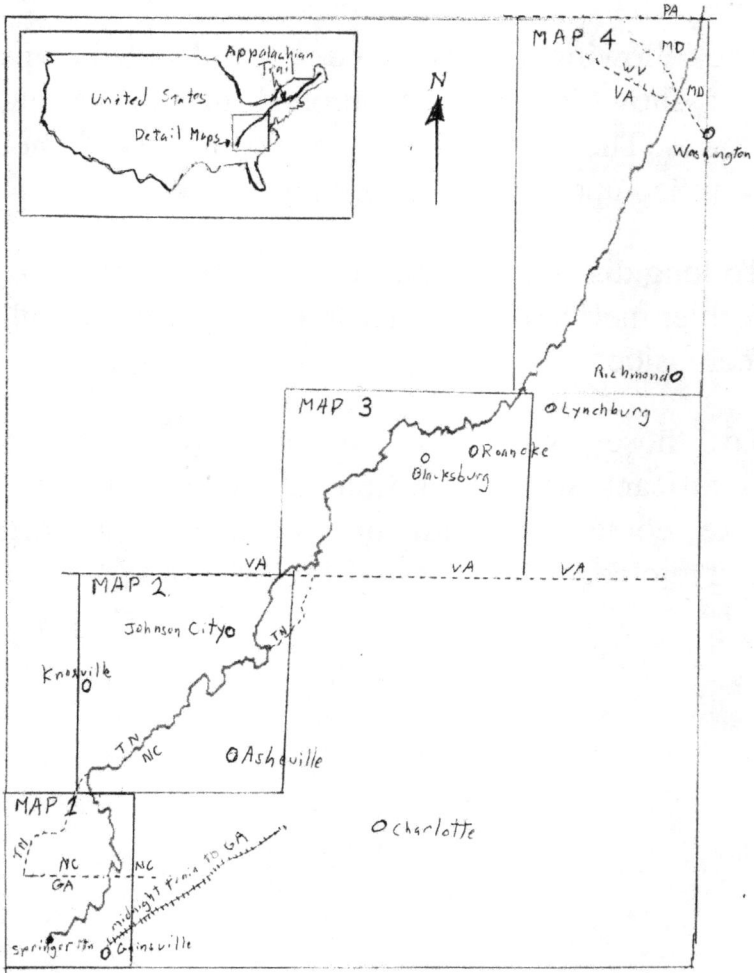

Map 1 - GA/NC

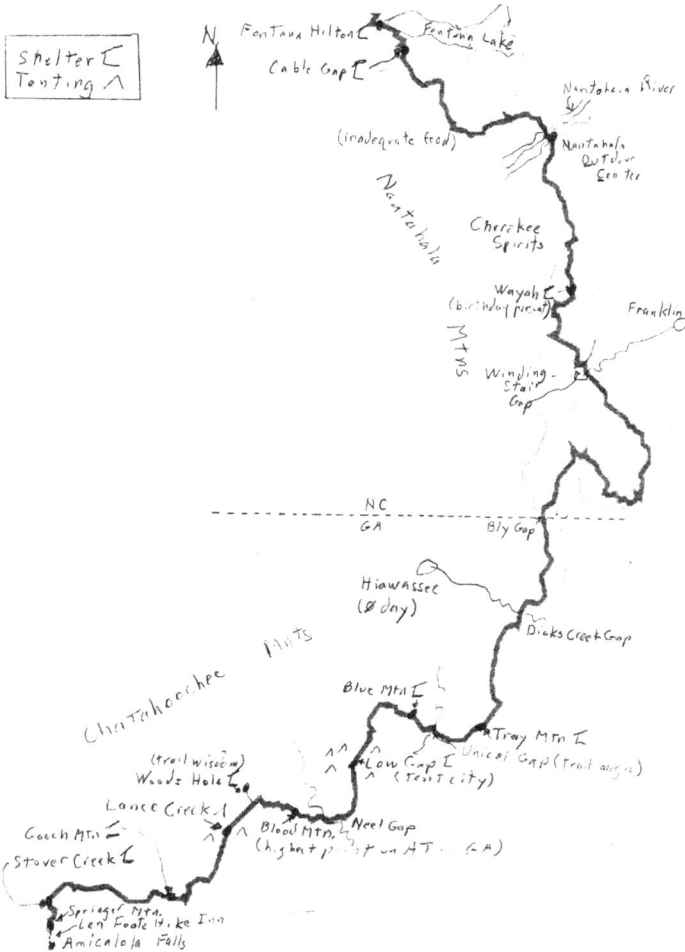

Beginning

April 23, 2012, Blue Mountain Shelter, GA

Finally, some time to write.

Monday, the train from NYC to Gainesville, GA. Cousin Bob met me in NYC, and we bought falafel from a vendor cart. It was good to see him, and actually good to be in NYC. What a contrast, yet it felt good.

As soon as I boarded the Crescent, I met Mary, sitting across the aisle. She lives in Peekskill, and was on her way to Birmingham to spend time with the family. She was convinced that I would starve to death when she heard what I intended to do. I don't think I've ever met anyone so generous. She kept throwing candy bars at me, showering me with food, and good wishes.

Tuesday – As it was getting lighter, I strained for a glimpse of the mountains, but could not see them at all. Then we moved into a thick fog as we approached Gainesville.

Ron was waiting for me right at the train door. He gave me a ride to the lodge, where I had my first grits of the hike. Then I grabbed my pack and poles, and started my adventure.

I headed down the steps, toward the falls, and was overcome with emotion. Yes, the falls are beautiful, but it was more than that. It was being in the mountains, and it was the beginning of living a dream. I called Jose and could barely speak.

I hiked down the falls, and back up with my pack. It was very hard work. I knew this was not going to be easy.

Then I started up the approach trail to the Len Foote Hike Inn. It was a perfect day, and I was enjoying it. While I was eating lunch, a group of 18 from Asheville came by and explained the new plants to me. They were impressed that I was beginning my thru hike.

The inn was a fantastic place, surrounded by gardens of native plants, and fabulous mountain views. The food was excellent, and sure tasted good after the climb up there. The dinner program about thru hiking really got me excited, since that is what I intended to do - hike the entire trail within 12 months.

Wednesday - The rain started
Tuesday night, and continued
steadily. It was warm, but
constant. Breakfast was fun.
Everyone was wishing me well. I
ate with the Texans, and they
asked me to let them know how I
make out.

As I boarded the Crescent in NYC, the conductor announced the list of stops through the South, ending in New Orleans. I did not know the South, but I would.

The train was a portal to another reality, a different reality, a reality that I would soon become a part of. It connected the confusion and abstraction of midtown NYC with... I knew not what. The speed and smoothness with which I sailed across the continent would become inconceivable to me only a few weeks later. I was on the midnight train to Georgia.

The A.T.'s rather unremarkable southern terminus is on top of Springer Mountain, in Georgia. That is mile 0. But before you can start hiking it, you have to get to it. Caveman said that it took him 2 days. For me, that included the walk along part of Amicalola Falls, the tallest cascading waterfall in the Southeast.

And, of course, the night spent at Len Foote Hike Inn, which is run by an affiliate of the Georgia Appalachian Mountain Club. It would be the last time I would sleep in a bed and eat real food for awhile. After dozing on the train the night before, and the hike up there, I truly enjoyed the amenities.

The A.T. is around 2200 miles, not road miles, trail miles, through the mountains. So it takes a substantial commitment of time, energy, and a bit of courage to contemplate a long distance hike. For many years trapped in a stale cubicle, I had been dreaming of this day. The feelings I had when I climbed the falls were incredibly intense. My first Appalachian Trail Moment (AT moment)!

My adventure was beginning.

Rain and Trail Wisdom

April 23, 2012, Blue Mountain Shelter, GA

***

And so I started my adventure in the rain. As I climbed, my glasses steamed up, and my poncho kept shifting. But it was ok. I knew it was the first rain, but surely not the last.

I got to the summit of Springer, and signed the register under the rock. It seemed so much smaller than I imagined. I was now at mile 0.

As I hiked toward the shelter near the summit, I passed a married couple and their young son, TyeDye. He asked if I was hiking the whole trail, and when I said "will see", he seemed impressed. Little did I know that we would be sharing a lot of time together.

I ate lunch in the shelter with an old man and his son and grandsons. We talked a bit. It was hard to understand their thick GA accents, plus the old man had a speech impediment.

I pushed on. After a bit, the rain stopped, but a thick fog moved in. I hiked to Stover Creek shelter, but was too tired to go on. That's where I met Indian Brave, 2 other hikers just starting out, and an experienced thru hiker, Trekking Pole, originally from Poland. It was going to be interesting.

Thursday - No rain, but very foggy. I enjoyed the hiking a lot, and had a very good day, going 13 miles to Gooch Mountain shelter. TyeDye and his family were there. I was tired, but felt like I was starting to get in better shape, and learn the ropes, or rather, the bear cables etc.

Friday - Well, the hiking went fine on a fabulous day. It was about 9 miles, but when I got to Lance Creek, all of the tent sites were taken. I found a spot at the end, and shared it with TyeDye and family.

But the mood was ominous. We were on the edge of extreme bear activity. There were many shots at nightfall, and someone said it was the rangers driving bears back. It was the first time setting up the tent, and rain was predicted. There were no bear cables, so we all struggled to make do. I was concerned that mine was not good, and that a bear could push the whole tree over. I slept fitfully in the tent.

Saturday – At the very first light, it began raining, and soon was a torrent. Water was pouring into the tent from the ground perimeter, (now I know what those little clips are for), and every big drop off the trees caused a little one inside. I tried to channel the rising flood inside the tent around the island of the sleeping pad. I moved the sleeping bag and down vest to the top to try to keep them dry, with some success.

But we had to break camp and move on. It was dismal: shitting in the woods in the driving rain, retrieving the food (thank goodness it was still there!), everything soaked thru the stuff sack, packing everything up, including the soaking tent. Every time I opened the pack to put something in, more rain poured in.

And then it was time to put on the soaked pack and march up Blood Mountain, the highest peak on the A.T. in GA. Because of the bear activity, the shelter was closed to overnight camping, so I would have to slog up and over to Neal Gap.

It was horrendous. The trail was a river with water falls. I met a group of 20 young men, I think they were military. We exchanged greetings and slogged on.

I knew I had to get into a shelter to change clothes. I was getting cold. It was raining too hard to do anything. Finally, I saw the sign for Woods Hole shelter. It was supposed to be .5 miles west, but it seemed like 5 miles to me.

Finally, I rounded the bend, and spotted it. An old man was sitting inside, reading a book with his head light on.

"What are you doing out there in a rain like this?", he asked. "Get in here."

I was only too eager to do just that. I took off the soaked clothes, and wrung them out. I dumped enough water out of my boots to fill a liter bottle. It was raining so hard and the pounding on the tin roof was so loud I could barely here him. But it began to let up, and we talked.

His name is Four Bears, and he is 80 years old, and on his second A.T. thru hike. That man imparted a lot of wisdom to me. On bear oder eliminating stuff sacks, on radios, on philosophy, on what it means to hike the A.T. "You will remember it the rest of your life because it is so hard", he said. At that moment, I knew he spoke the truth.

And then, miraculously, the rain stopped and the sun began to poke through. He suggested I reserve a cabin at Neal Gap to dry out. We had a good signal, so I did. Glad I did.

So I bid him farewell, and continued on, in much better shape. The hike to the top of Blood Mountain was easier than I thought, and when I got there, TyeDye and his family were there. I took pictures of them, and we enjoyed the views.

Heading down to Neal Gap was fairly easy, but the rocks were slippery. When I got there, the whole crew was there. They cheered me on.

I headed over to the cabins, signed in, and bought a large pizza and coke. I took a luxurious shower. And I began drying everything out, including the tent in the bathtub. I uploaded pictures, ate pizza, and slept very well.

TyeDye was an inspiration to me. He was only 7 years old, and was carrying all of his food. He was experiencing the same difficult conditions and walking the same miles we all were, but with less complaining, and a lot more energy. I thought about him often as I made my way north.

Most of the time, I tried to make it to a shelter to spend the night. There are over 250 shelters on the A.T. that can be used by hikers on a first-come, first-served basis. The shelters are usually a floor with 3 walls and a roof, open on the front. As the name implies, they are shelter from the rain and wet ground. And shelters are usually located near a water source, an essential ingredient of life.

What makes a shelter memorable? Many, different things. How about a stone fireplace, right inside? Or maybe a private penthouse on the third level. What about dovetail joints in a log structure, so that it is built like a fine piece of furniture? Maybe it's perched up on a narrow ridge, like a watch tower, or situated for the perfect sunrise or sunset. You will remember that gusher of a spring, right in the front yard. Maybe it's the possibility of food delivery direct to your virtual door, or the spectacularly clean and fresh privy. Sometimes it's the things you might rather not remember, like the snake under the floor. Many reasons to remember a shelter.

If a shelter was too far to reach or was full, I relied on my tent. It was an extremely light weight tent with no rain fly, so it was not particularly well suited to the wet conditions of the Appalachian Trail. Sure, it's important that your equipment is light weight. But you really can't discount it's primary function - to try to keep you dry.

Well, I sure did get acquainted with rain while I was living outside: warm rain, cold rain, scary, hypothermia inducing rain.

Rain, even warm, gentle rain, has a way of seeping right into you, physically and emotionally. Rain brings the water we need to live, and the pain of penetrating cold.

And really, you have to surrender to rain. Oh sure, there are all sorts of "water proof" garments, but still, in a driving, all day, heavy rain, you will be wet. You try to get used to it.

Trail wisdom says that you should never decide to end your hike on a rainy day. Good advice. The temptation to be warm and dry is enormous. Caveman points out that this is very good advice for life in general. Save it for a sunny day.

Trekking Pole was the first experienced hiker I met on the trail. I was astonished when he said that thru hikers were lazy. "How can that be"?, I asked. You mean someone who is hiking over 2000 miles is lazy? I did not know then, but I now understand that it takes so much energy to hike 2000 miles, that you will conserve every ounce that you can, otherwise, it might well be impossible. So, when he looked at my supplies, he gently pointed out that I could live for a long time in the mountains with what he saw in my pack. At the same time, I was surprised to see how little he had in his. But he knew what he was doing. I did not.

Gradually, we were acquiring our own trail wisdom. Most of the shelters in GA are equipped with bear cables in the back yard. The concept is to hang your food bag on a line which is suspended above a bear's reach. When we were camping away from a shelter, there were no bear cables, so we needed to improvise our own. The goal is to hang your bag from a limb far enough out from the trunk so it would be out of reach of the bears. Mine that night was terrible, a bear probably could have pushed the whole tree over.

And pretty quickly, I learned how to do a better job of setting up my tent. And most important, don't wear cotton, which turns into a heavy, cold mess when it gets wet. And so on. It felt good later in my hike to be able to help other, less experienced hikers by sharing what I learned. We helped each other out.

Cold

April 23, 2012, Blue Mountain
Shelter, GA

***

Sunday — Ate 2 egg and cheese
biscuits, packed up, and moved
out. I stopped at the outfitters at
Neal Gap and bought a smell
proof stuff sack, fuel, and some
food. I dropped the old stuff
sack in the hiker box and
continued up the trail.

It was a fabulous day, cool and
bright. The trail was gorgeous,
with sunny ledges to stop and
enjoy fabulous views all the way.
But I wanted to get to Low Gap
shelter because I knew the whole
crew would be there, and it was
really the next shelter on the A.T.

While I was resting, a hiker from

Nashville came up. We walked together for a long way. I really pushed because I knew it would be tough to get to Low Gap shelter, but we did it. Got in just before dark. And it was COLD!

It was an entire tent city. At least 17, and the shelter full. So I set up my tent. Fortunately, it was dry. I cooked on the ground, and then I socialized at the two campfires.

Indian Brave was at the second one, along with Medicine Man. We smoked and talked about all kinds of stuff, from quantum physics to mushrooms. Medicine Man has a way with getting the fire to burn. I think he does it with pure energy.

I turned in, and submerged into my sleeping bag. It was cold and windy, but I was ok, and slept well.

Well, that brings me up to date. Indian Brave just arrived, so I'm going to go join him and do some cooking. Frost predicted for tonight, so I'll cook 2 packages of Ramen with all the fixings.

April 26, Hiawassee, GA

COLD! That was the word on Monday. It was very cold up there on aptly named Blue Mountain. We were all turning blue. I made the mistake of not putting on two pairs of socks, so I had to curl into a fetal position to sleep, but eventually I did.

Tuesday — Ate oatmeal, and walked from Blue Mountain shelter to Tray Mountain, 8.1 miles. It was a gorgeous day, and a gorgeous walk, despite the cold winds, with views everywhere.

When I got down to Unicoi Gap, a trail angel, Dr. Pepper, appeared. He offered me a Dr. Pepper soda, and a bag of various trail treats that powered me to Hiawassee.

Neal Gap is the first major milestone you encounter on the A.T. as you head north. It is around 32 miles north of Springer Mountain, so by now you have a pretty good idea of what the A.T. is like, and what you are up against. It seems inconceivable that you have only walked 32 miles, after so much effort. It is a major road crossing, with a hiker hostel, and a good place to quit. Some do.

Only later did I grasp what I had been told by the outfitters at Neal Gap. They offer a free service to go through your pack with you, to identify stuff you will not need and should mail back home. I declined the service. After all, I was an experienced hiker after hiking many sections of the A.T. When I bought the fuel for my heavy cooking stove, they said, "Going heavy, aren't you". After carrying that stove for 1000 miles, I now know that they were correct. But they were wrong about the size of the food sack to buy. I eat twice as much as most hikers.

Dr. Pepper was the first trail angel I encountered on the trail. He was parked at the road crossing at Unicoi Gap, and had a cooler full of cold soda, and bags of candy treats that he was giving out to hikers. It was always a pleasure to encounter a cooler with cold drinks at road crossings. One time, it was a day hiker who gave me a half dozen Krispy Creme doughnuts, squashed into a sticky mass that I scarfed down. We were on a pilgrimage of sorts, and appreciated the kindness of strangers. Many of them were motivated by christian values of giving, especially to travelers in the wilderness. I am indebted to them all.

It was mid April in GA. But we were hiking between 3000 and 4000 feet. Like rain, cold penetrates. And the need to keep our pack weight down means we skimp on clothes. Socks become gloves, and a sleeping bag is salvation.

Try to imagine how good those campfires felt. Our little encampment was hearth and home, just then.

Zero Mile Days and Food

April 26, Hiawassee, GA

***

Wednesday - I decided to hike from Tray Mountain shelter all the way to Dick's Creek Gap. Rain was predicted, and so it made sense to shoot for Hiawassee to dry out, resupply, and take a 0 mile day. It was a long day, 11 miles. There was just one mountain. But as I walked down to the gap, I was exhausted. I knew I needed a 0 day.

When I got to the gap, Indian Brave, Crossfit, and Mandy were sitting at a picnic table, and another hiker was trying to hitch. After trying for an hour, he did not have any luck. It seemed that there was not a signal up there. Finally, Indian Brave was able to get through, and 45 minutes later, we were all packed into a jeep, Mandy on my lap.

We pulled into town, hallucinating food the whole way. We went to the "all you can eat" Chinese buffet right after we checked in, and then to Dairy Queen for banana splits. And then we all got together to relax, smoke, and talk.

Thursday - Our first zero mile day, Wow! I really like zero mile days. A vacation from the vacation.

Started out by going over to the South Side Cafe for breakfast. Three eggs, sausage, home fries and grits and toast. Everyone was so friendly. At least 4 people came over to say hello, and to urge me to be careful.

The waitress said she just got a text message warning about T-storms. And then it started to pour, and then quarter sized hail. She said her father would take me back to the Budget Inn when it slowed down. It did slow down, and I made a run for it.

We hung out, and then Indian Brave and I went for lunch and groceries. We did laundry. And then all the hikers gathered on the porch to gossip and compare blisters, smoke, eat, laugh and live. It felt good.

Tomorrow, we head back up to the mountains, and I can't wait. I feel rested and ready.

I was 63 when I hiked those 1000 miles. I really did need those zero mile days, even though no miles of the A.T. were accomplished. Days spent in town eating, cleaning up, eating, fixing equipment, eating, charging phone, eating, food shopping, eating...

Some hikers eschew zero days in town, but most do avail themselves of the amenities. Before my hike, I did not really understand how much a part of the experience days in town would be. It was a way to get to know the natives, and what the South really is.

On the trail, we all hallucinate food. For me, smells, mostly. My mind can conjure a plausible Chinese buffet fragrance. Oh, how we suffered.

You burn maybe 5000 calories a day hiking the trail. Go ahead, just try to see how much food you have to carry for 5000 calories per day. And how heavy is that? Bottom line for most of us - slow starvation. Pretty intense.

And rest. Give those sore joints and muscles a day off. Cut off the old blisters. And sleep on a bed, with real sheets.

But, curiously, at the end of the 0, itching to get back on the trail. Why? Was it the cleaner air, the views, the animals? We were beginning our intense attraction to the trail, and it was pulling on us. Rain and cold be dammed!

And so, we all piled onto the back of a pickup truck, and breezed through the mountains, hair blowing in the slip stream. We were free, heading back to the trail we love, our new home.

Hikers

May 2, Franklin NC

Well, I'm giving up now on a day by day journal. The shelters are beginning to merge into one another. The trail way of life is becoming routine now, but not the experiences. So I'll concentrate on the perceptions and feelings instead.

People — This is the first topic, since it has been the most significant. Our little group has solidified into a family, and we are helping each other out so much.

Test Run — Louisiana/Virginia Beach. veteran of the Afghanistan war, PETA officer. Lives in his RV, retired military, early 40's.

Slaughter House — Kansas, 23,

vegetarian eating meat on the trail. Wants to go to DC after the trail, and then the Peace Corps.

Bambi - Knoxville TN, 57, retired from the TVA. Very dry sense of humor. Pushing on, enjoying the torture of the journey.

#5 & Zen - Rangeley ME. Young, cute couple. She is an RN, administering to us all.

Indian Brave - Boston, 24, gorgeous young hunk, 6'2", huge calves and legs, marathon runner.

The trail - Getting into NC was quite a trip. It sure felt good crossing that first state line. But what a climb up out of Bly Gap! Mountains here are bigger, 5500 feet, with gaps down around 4000 feet. The leaves are not out at all on top, so there is a lot more sun than I expected. There are whole hillsides of trilliums in full bloom. The trail is mercifully not as steep as in GA, and we are in better shape now, but it is still a bit of a struggle for me on the ups.

The youthful vigor of the trail – These are some of the oldest mountains in the world, but the power and strength of youth is everywhere present. The predominate age seems to be early 20's. But there are people like Take 5 who is 70, and Four Bears who is 80. And me. I have to say, it does give me a good feeling to be hiking with the kids. I know I can't really keep up, but hey, I'm very pleased with how I'm doing. And it sure makes me feel younger. Our shared trials and tribulations do bond us together, no matter our ages. I don't think there are too many other places where that is as true.

Our second 0 day was in Franklin, and how we did enjoy it. On our last afternoon in town, we all gathered at a bar, and met up with 2 older women hikers from Texas and Georgia. We were all from different states, so the bar simply labeled our tabs with our state name. Our stories were from our different homes, and of course, our new home, the trail.

The bonds that form among long distance hikers grow incredibly strong. We are on the trail a long time with each other. It takes time.

We take care of each other. #5 attended to our cuts, scrapes, and intestinal issues. When it was dry, we shared water. When equipment broke, we pitched in to fix it.

This practice of taking care of each other was even more intense with the veterans of wars like Test Run. He presented me with a container of his special Louisiana hot spice that I relied on for the rest of my hike. So many of the vets really did watch your back, literally, as we walked north. That "keeping an eye on you" practice was true for most hikers, but even more so with the vets. I wished that I could have imparted the peace of a good night's sleep that so many of them found illusive.

Indian Brave was the first millennial that I got to really know. We did a lot of talking about an idea of his. He wanted to apply techniques he knew about to help people read faster and better from mobile devices. In the bromance that later developed, we co-founded a company to pursue some of those ideas. But that is another story.

I did not know it at the time, but Bambi and I were becoming trail buddies. We were both about the same age, and hiked about the same number of miles every day, and our temperaments were compatible. I loved his dry sense of sometimes black humor.

Trail lore says that many hikers drop out before even getting out of GA. I remember Bambi proudly announcing that it would never be him. Then he stepped across the state line, and said, "Ok, now I can quit." Of course he kept going.

A Gift We Accept Gratefully

May 10, Fontana Hilton Shelter

It's been awhile since Franklin, and some tough hiking. The hike from Franklin, climbing up out of the photogenic Winding Stair Gap to the Nantahala Outdoor Center went ok at first. Bambi and I kept up with Test Run, Slaughter, #5 and Zen. Pulled into the shelter with rain gushing down.

But that was the last time I saw them for awhile. They were definitely going faster than Bambi and I. And the rain continued. We went slowly.

We decided to book into the hostel at the Nantalala Outdoor Center. We got to the gorge in bright sun, with everyone cavorting in the river. We showered and headed to the restaurant.

And joy! There they were! The whole group! Test Run, Slaughter, #5 and Zen. So we moved into the corner table outside by the river, and ate and drank. It was so good to be with them.

The hike out of the Nantalala Outdoor Center started out fine, considering the steep climb. But the next day was one of the worst. The trail was tough - a lot of up and down, and we were tired. We both felt that we were loosing physical strength. The re-supply at NOC was completely inadequate. I had 1 stale bagel, a stack of Ritz crackers, some peanut butter and honey, and that was it for lunch food. But we could not eat even that, because of the rain.

Rain. Hard driving rain. Torrents of it. I could not manage to get my poncho on, so I just stood there in it, watching it pour down the trail. I looked like some unfortunate cow, staring down at the ground, water cascading off my body.

The next day was quite nice - no rain. Cable Gap shelter was beautiful and quiet. An old, log style small shelter with a stream in the front yard. Bambi and I got in early, maybe 3:30. We enjoyed a nice, easy rest in a beautiful spot.

Yesterday, Bambi and I hiked in a light rain all day. Down, down. down. Slipping, sliding, slogging down the slimy trail.

But then we slid into the Fontana Marina, and were soon teleported to what we were dreaming of: a hot shower, good food, laundry, and resupply. It was good, but somehow we missed the trail. Strange. It is very nice, and we look forward to it, but it is an alien world to us now.

So here I sit at the picnic table in front of the Fontana Hilton, in the sun. I took a dip in the lake - it was great. And this morning, Bambi and I took a tour of the dam. He seemed nostalgic for his TVA job. And as much as we are enjoying this wonderful day here, we are both itching to hit the trail again. Trail madness? I don't know. I guess it's what we do now. Hike.

***

It was quite a raucous crowd of musicians here last night. They got a nice fire going, and invited

us down to enjoy it. And then
someone I did not even know
starting tossing beers to us all,
which I gratefully accepted.

They got out an iPhone app to
tune up the compact guitar, and
the banjo, and the music stated.
The guitar player performed a
song he was writing about the A.T.
It spoke of the freedom of
knowing that everything you need
is on your back. The images were
real and vivid. The song was
intense, especially heard that way,
around the campfire with a bunch
of vagabonds.

Earlier today, Bambi and I were
looking at a model of the A.T. at
the visitors center. Now you can
actually see the part we have
hiked. The Chattahoochee
National Forest, and now the
Nantahala (noon day sun)
mountains.

Soon we will begin on the Smokies. We flow through the country, foot by foot, and sense how the accents change, how the landscape changes, how the mountains change. It is a gift we accept gratefully. So let us continue.

The trail bestows many gifts. The Fontana Hilton, actually named the Fontana Shelter, is one. It has running water, and a shower and toilet nearby. Believe me, those are gifts to a long distance hiker.

And then there was the birthday gift I unexpectedly received the day after we left Franklin. When I pulled into Wayah Shelter, Slaughter House presented me with an icy cold beer that she carried all the way up there. I offered it around, but of course no one would take so much as a sip of my birthday present. A birthday to remember.

But not all of the gifts are so pleasant. I have vivid memories of a cold, misty day in the

Nantahalas, as I trudged through the fog. I was thinking about the Cherokee people who lived here before they were evicted. Suddenly, I was overcome by a deep cold, more penetrating even than on the coldest days. I think I was feeling their pain and sadness.

And the trail bestows knowledge, too. It was teaching Bambi and I how our bodies worked, or didn't work. We learned about food, and what our bodies needed to keep going. When was the optimal time to consume that snickers bar, based on the miles to go, and the elevation change. And most of all, that influenced our re-supply for the rest of the trip.

But the trail beckoned. What's up ahead? What is the land like? The trees? The water? The people? We were flowing through the mountains, foot by foot, and grateful for the days, rain or shine.

Map 2 - Smokies

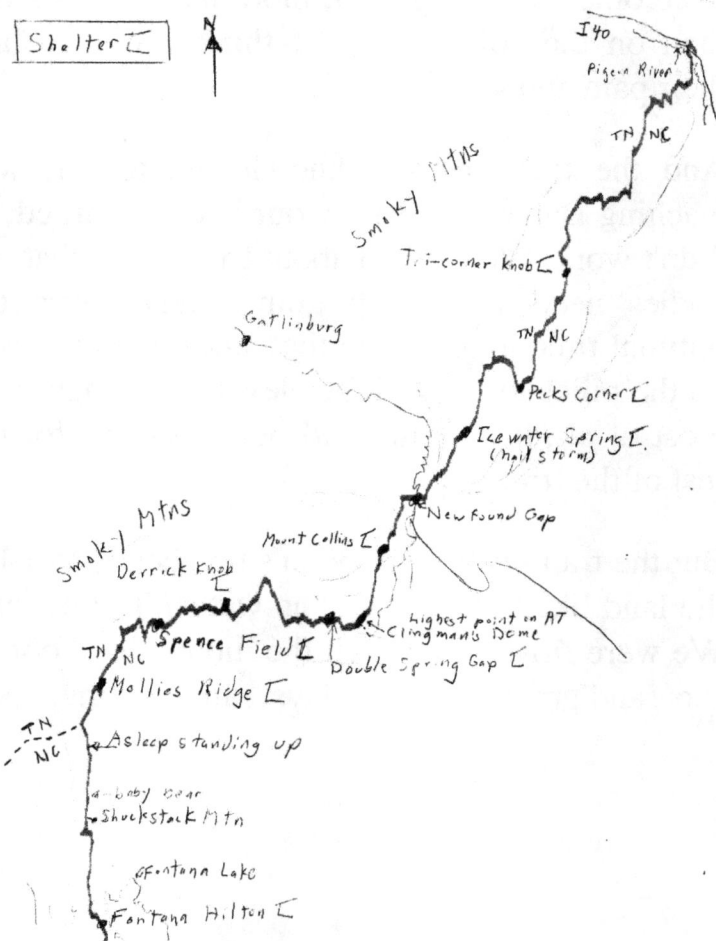

Shelter ⊏

N

I 40
Pigeon River

TN NC

Smoky Mtns

Tri-corner knob ⊏

TN NC

Gatlinburg

Pecks Corner ⊏

Ice water Spring ⊏
(hail storm)

New Found Gap

Smoky Mtns

Mount Collins ⊏

Derrick Knob ⊏

highest point on AT
Clingmans Dome

TN
NC   Spence Field ⊏

Double Spring Gap ⊏

Mollies Ridge ⊏

TN
NC

Asleep standing up

baby bear
Shuckstack Mtn

Fontana Lake

Fontana Hilton ⊏

48

Asleep Standing Up

May 12, Spence Field, Smoky
Mountains National Park

I'm sitting here in a field of lush,
green grass, with some scrub trees
around the edge. My pack is
leaning against one of the trees,
and I'm seated on the grass,
leaning up against it. The sun is
poking through the clouds at
times, and at other times, the
clouds are thick. The wind is
alternately cresting strong, and
then subsiding almost completely.

I hiked here with Bambi from
Mollies Ridge shelter. It was an
easy walk, maybe 6 miles, and I
am grateful to be here.

On the way over, we met a ridge
runner. He asked if we were ok, if
we had filled out a permit, and
when we started at Springer. Then

he informed us that there was a 40% chance of showers today, 60% tonight, and 100% tomorrow. He told us to prepare to get wet.

Well, for sure, we knew it would be almost impossible not to get wet. So we will get wet. So what?

We decided to stay at the shelter near here because the next stretch, to Derrick Knob shelter, would be tough. It's around 2 pm, and we just did not want to push on.

I'm so glad I'm here, and so glad for the short day again. What a beautiful spot.

What a contrast from yesterday. That was the toughest day yet for me, tougher than anything else since Springer. It was only 11.5 miles, but a climb of 4000 feet!

The climb went ok at first. After all, we were rested, fresh from the Fontana Hilton. I was hiking by myself. I came to the side trail to Shuckstack Mountain. Wasn't sure what it was, so glad I checked. It was not far to the fire tower, so I went up to it.

Well, what a great place for lunch. I gingerly ascended the weathered stairs. The top was open, so I went in. The view was breathtaking! 360 degrees. The dam, Fontana Village, the marina, and the lake most of the way to Wesser. In the background were the Nantahala Mountains. No wonder they were so steep. They looked incredibly rugged.

And then I turned around to behold the Smokies. Yikes! Bigger yet, and more rugged. And that ribbing on the sides, like you see on the model at the Fontana Dam visitors center.

After lunch, I headed down from the tower, and met an older couple from Alabama. They hiked all the way up there for the view. That is an incredible climb for the view. I bid them farewell and headed back down to the A.T.

And then, in less than a quarter mile, I heard a scampering in the woods about 10 feet away up the trail. I turned, and saw the cutest live teddy bear, maybe 2 feet long, looking back at me. I really wanted to stop and get a picture, but I knew that mama bear was nearby, so I kept walking. But it was such a privilege to see that bear. I hope it's not the last one I see.

Seeing that baby bear cub was a true gift, and there were other bear stories. I remember a ranger telling us about a smart mama bear training her cub to steal hiker food in the Smokies. She would send the cub toward the shelter. Once all the hikers were distracted, she would rummage through any unwatched packs.

Encountering a ridge runner, or anyone acting in an official capacity, is a fairly rare experience on the A.T. We were hiking in heavily visited Great Smoky Mountains National Park. The ridge runners are there to keep an eye on the trail, and not to support hikers. But on most of the trail, you are really on your own. There are no guard rails on the A.T.

But the Smokies can be tough. First, you have to get up into them. I can now say, it was the toughest day for me ever on the trail. I enjoyed the climb, but was completely exhausted toward the end. My hiking buddies scratched encouraging messages into the mud with their walking sticks. "Will See, you can do it!" It helped.

Unless you have experienced that kind of exhaustion, you will not understand, or believe this. But I once fell asleep standing up, leaning against a tree, with my fully loaded backpack on. A passing hiker woke me up to make sure I was still alive.

Tough Days in the Smokies

May 15, Gatlinburg TN

Wow, what a couple of days I have just lived through! Barely.

The night at Spence Field was very pleasant. The rain started, but we were quite cozy. The local guys brought some good rum which they shared with us. We enjoyed that, and swapped stories.

But the evening was permeated with thoughts of the next day. The prediction was for cold, heavy rain. It was ominous. We were not let down.

All night, the rain pelted the roof. And by morning, it was torrential. So we did breakfast, put on ponchos, and headed out into it.

At first it did not seem too bad, now that we could no longer hear it pounding on the tin roof. When we went across the peaks of Thunderhead, the blowing mist seemed quite mysterious and beautiful. It compensated somewhat for not having a view.

As I moved along, I saw another baby bear scurry into the rhododendrons, second siting so far.

But as we trudged on, the rain and wind picked up and the trail got muddier. It got colder, with temperatures in the 40's. My poncho was blowing up in my face. I had to look over my completely steamed up glasses to try to see. The wind was so strong on the peaks we could barely stand.

And then, as I semi-blindly crawled along, there was a deep growl just ahead on the trail. It really startled me. But before I could even stop, a big bear moved off the trail into the bushes.

It was a long, slow muddy slog. I fell twice. The second time, I tobogganed down the muddy slope on my backpack. It was exhausting. Because of the rain, we could not stop, so I was getting a little weak from hunger. I was munching on trail food, but even that was difficult because my hands, and everything else, were covered in mud. It was only 6.5 miles to Derrick Knob shelter, but it seemed to take forever.

Finally, there it was. It was already pretty full of cold, wet hikers. Lines of dripping clothes were everywhere. I finally ate lunch, got into dry clothes, and got into my sleeping bag. After awhile, I warmed up, got out, and made a big dinner. We all commiserated about how close we had come to experiencing hypothermia. It was one of the most difficult days of my life, but it was over.

The next day was a lot better. It was 5.5 miles to Siler's Bald shelter. The rain stopped, and it was warmer, but the trail was a mud slide. We got to the shelter and had lunch.

We started out for Double Spring Gap shelter, but turned back when it started to rain. It stopped, so we started again, then more rain, so we returned yet again. Finally, on the third attempt, we just kept going when the rain started, and arrived without incident. It was pretty full, but there was room. We settled in and made dinner.

Then, not much before dark, two young women showed up and moved in. They said there would be 6 more of the boys coming soon. Well, that put us 2 over capacity. They were young and had met on the trail, but seemed pretty close. And with a military air, but friendly, too.

But it was horrendous. They and their stuff were everywhere. All they wanted to talk about was how many miles they were doing, and it was a lot! We were so crammed in on the upper deck that my head lamp was under my neighbors body. Trying to get down to pee in the middle of the night was not so easy, but we managed.

The next morning, it was a tower of babel of confusion, so I stayed in my sleeping bag as long as possible. And finally, they started leaving, and we were able to eat and get going.

We hiked the 3 miles and 1100 feet up to Clingman's Dome, the highest point on the A.T. It went pretty easily. As we got up there, we got into the firs. It was nice to be in an alpine environment.

We got to the tower, but everything was socked in. As we sat at the bottom, several people came over to talk. They seemed amused/astonished/confused when we said we had walked from GA, and intended to walk to Maine. We enjoyed the interaction with the civilians.

Because there were no views, we decided to go down to the parking lot to see if we could get a ride out, and come back up another day. A ranger came over and said that a taxi was in the lot, and asked if we wanted a ride down. We jumped at the chance.

The ride down was spectacular, the mountains huge. I overflowed with emotion.

And then we were in Gatlinburg, very honky-tonk, very strange. But still, it was nice to be in "civilization" again. Good food, and free moonshine.

Three million people use the A.T. every year. Some are not hikers at all, and simply come for the views and clean air. Others are day hikers, and drive to a convenient road crossing, hike for a few miles, or do some sort of loop hike, returning to the car before evening. Section hikers take on a section of the trail that they hike in a few days, weeks, or months. Usually they are prepared to sleep up in the mountains, on the trail. Thru hikers attempt to hike the entire trail within 12 months.

One of the day hikers aptly renamed the Smokies the Soakies. Views were lacking because we were socked in so much of the time. I did not fully connect with the Smokies until later.

Gatlinburg was a respite for us. It was not like the other trail towns, being much bigger, and a tourist destination. Dolly Wood was not very far away. A legal moonshine operator offered free samples to those old enough to drink. Gatlinburg got us out of the rain and the cold for awhile, and we surely enjoyed that, too.

But the shelters in the Smokies were to die for (hopefully not). They were built by the Civilian Conservation Corps in the 1930's, and constructed of stone. There was usually a large, double sleeping deck with a skylight. And best of all, there was a fireplace in the shelter. Try to imagine how cozy it was that night at Spence Field Shelter up there on the mountain, trading stories with the local kids around the fire as the rain pounded the roof.

Heroes

I'm sitting in the sun, and it sure feels good. My boots are in the sun, and socks hanging in a tree in the sun to dry. It's mid afternoon. We decided to just come here from Icewater Spring shelter, around 7.5 miles. It was just too far to go close to double that, and I've become very comfortable with our pace through the Smokies.

Rainbow is here. We met him back at Icewater Spring shelter. His feet are bad, so he just came here.

Day before yesterday, we took the taxi from Gatlinburg to Clingman's Dome. We felt pretty good passing all the civilians as we made our way up that .5 mile road with our full packs on. When we got up there, surprise, there was Candy Cane. He was so shocked to see us, that he caught up to us. He was heading out to Knoxville to earn money for a couple of weeks. I wonder if/when we will see him again?

The view from the tower was spectacular, but a little anti-climactic. Of course, I tried to take some pictures, but how can you capture that?

We headed back to the A.T., glad to be on the trail again. It was good to be among the huge firs, even if they were dying. How spectacular it must have been 40 years ago.

We spent the night at the Mount Collins shelter. Two former (and current) thru hikers were there. They shared a lot of thoughts about thru hikers. One reason they might do it multiple times is because they are heroes doing it, but working at the local Xtra Mart when they get back, they are just regular people again.

Bambi later pointed out that these kids have the persistence, wisdom, and courage to be running things in 30 years. But will they? Does our culture recognize that? Maybe that's why things are the way they are.

Yesterday, we hiked down to New Found Gap and up to Icewater Spring shelter. When we got to the gap, a lot of civilians came over to chat, including the 80 year old guy who originally came from Holland. He had also been a park ranger, and seemed to miss that life.

We headed back up the trail. Rain was threatening, but I was hungry.

Once I was out of sight of the gap, I pulled out my lunch stuff, and it immediately started to rain. I huddled under my poncho, doing my best to create and eat lunch. Then it was slogging up the mountain, being wet inside and out.

After awhile, it stopped, and by the time I got to the shelter, it was just foggy. But within a few minutes, all hell broke loose, with torrential rain and tons of pea sized hail. It sure was good to be in that shelter.

Before very long, a bunch of day hikers began to pour in. I offered a shivering women a shirt, but she declined. It poured and poured and poured. Finally, it stopped, and they all left.

While I was walking along today, I had a thought. I really like the

natural world, and do well in it.
I feel good, eat well, sleep well,
am relaxed, and feel no tension.

All of this is somewhat curious.
How can I be more relaxed if it is
life threatening if I don't have
water or warm clothes? If I can
fall off a cliff or be struck by
lightening? Sure, it can be very
unpleasant, but I never feel the
anxiety that I feel in the
artificial world. It is becoming
clear to me that when my hike
ends, I need to be in the natural
world as much as possible.
Organic farmer? Makes sense.
Software engineer? I don't think
so.

It was so sad to see those towering, dead firs.
Most of them above 5000 feet are dead or dying.
The culprit was and is acid rain from burning
coal. Bambi said that it is a lot cleaner than it
used to be. But it's too late now. The pain of
seeing so much death up there will stay in my
memory forever.

Candy Cane was the source of quite a bit of concern on the trail. He had been seen by many, struggling up the trail in soaked jeans, dangerously ill-equipped. He came from the heart of Appalachia, but lacked the means to safely undertake such a journey. But he persisted bravely, and learned what he needed from us all, and taught us even more. It was an inspiration to us that he made it to the highest point on the A.T.

We had been on the trail about a month, and had hiked 217 miles. By now, we were quite fit. It sure felt good to pass all those civilians going up to Clingman's Dome. And then there was all the attention we got at New Found Gap. We felt like heroes.

But the trail was not done with us yet. Beware, pride comes before a fall.

Trail Names

May 20, Tri Corner Knob shelter

Easy day today, only 5.5 miles, and that has been a blessing. We had time to stop and look and listen. Finally, I think I am absorbing the Smokies, and they are beautiful. Yesterday, Bambi and I spent a lot of time at an overlook. The clouds were rolling up from deep below the cliff, getting caught up on the currents and blowing through the gap. The multiple layers of fog were moving in different directions, and the sun was shining through it all. Finally, I see and feel the beauty in these mountains. Yes, they are more than rain and hail and cold. They are gorgeous, and fill me with emotion.

Last night, Bambi and I were talking about how he has a knack for finding caves to hide in when it rains, so we agreed that henceforth, he shall be known as Caveman. He said his family would be amused.

The shelter here is beautiful. We are up high, so it's cool. The spring is right in the front yard. Rainbow is using my stove to cook our red beans and rice, and I will eat soon, and sleep well, as usual.

Eventually, almost every long distance hiker has a trail name. The name often evolves from some behavior or characteristic that is siezed upon by the local hiking community. For example, at the very beginning of the trail in GA, whenever anyone asked me a question I did not really know the answer to, I would reply, "Will See". How far are you going? Will See. Where are you camping tonight? Will See.

Candy Cane acquired his trail name at the Amicalola Falls visitor center when he stocked up on surplus candy canes they were giving away.

Trekking Pole's name had a double meaning: the walking sticks that we use are called "trekking poles", and he was from Poland, so it was a natural trail name for him.

Bambi and I had been hiking together, on and off, for about 3 weeks, so we were getting to know each other on the trail. I was really impressed by his ability to find shelter from the rain. I got used to finding him relaxing under a huge, downed tree, completely dry, or sitting under a rock overhang enjoying a dry break, while I was soaked to the skin. So "we", the local hiking community, changed his name to Caveman.

It could be worse, and often is. If the name fits, it will stick, and it is how you will be known, both verbally, and in the written trail logs that pass along news and gossip.

Some shorter distance hikers resist the whole thing, but this is not a good idea. So an inappropriately named hiker "John" becomes "Just John" when he continually insisted that his name was just John.

Almost every shelter has a trail log. A notebook and pen or pencil is enclosed in a plastic bag, and contained in some sort of box to prevent it from being eaten by wildlife or hungry hikers. Most hikers write an entry to document their passage. It usually contains the date, (as nearly as can be determined, since time seems to slip away on the trail), and information about the hike to the shelter. Often, there are graphic sketches to illustrate the text, and some are quite elaborate and beautiful. Hikers rely on information in the logs to learn about trail conditions on the other side of the shelter. Is there water where it should be? Any blowdowns (downed trees across the trail)? Was it a steep climb? Were wet rocks involved? And where is Sherlock?

Trail logs have existed on the A.T. for as long as there have been shelters. Even now, in the age of cell phones, they still are the most trusted, reliable and available source of information. Relying on cell phones solely is not a good idea on most of the trail. You might get enough of a signal to send a text at the top of a mountain, but paper and pencil work anywhere.

Map 3 - NC/TN

Shelter [

N

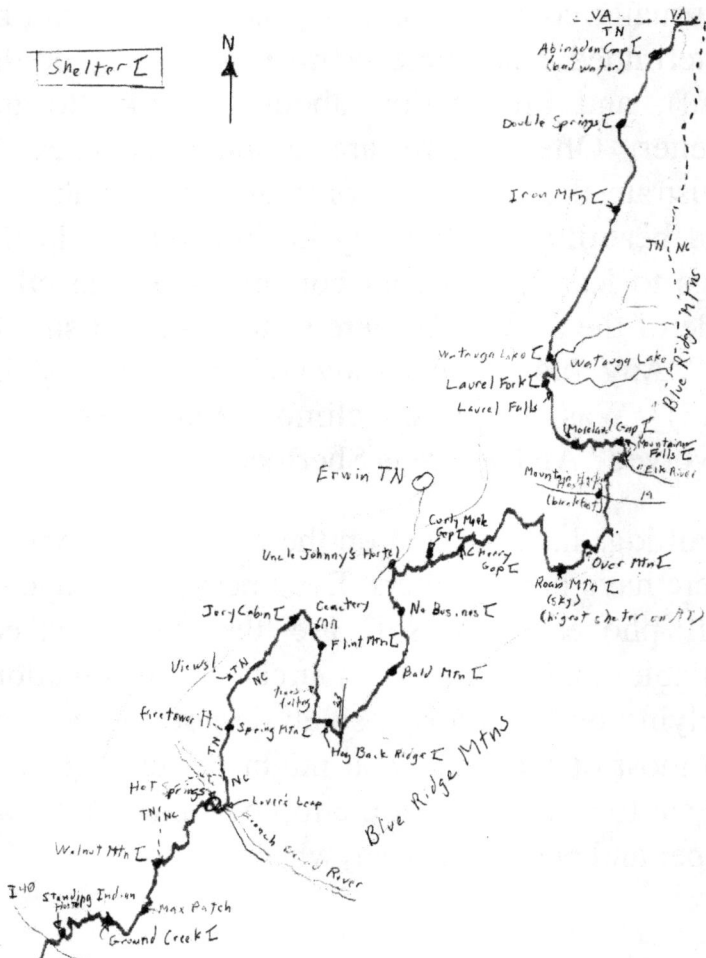

VA
TN
Abingdon Cap [
(end water)

VA

Double Springs [

Iron Mtn [

TN NC

Watauga Lake [
Laurel Fork [
Laurel Falls

Watauga Lake

Moreland Gap [

Mountaineer
Falls [
Elk River

Erwin TN

Mountain Harbor
Hostel
(breakfast)

Curly Maple
Gap [

Uncle Johnny's Hostel

NC Henry
Gap [

Over Mtn [

Roan Mtn [
(sky)
(highest shelter on AT)

Jerry Cabin [

Cemetery
600

No Business [

Views! TN
NC
Jerry
Valley

Flint Mtn [

Bald Mtn [

Firetower H

Spring Mtn [

Hog Back Ridge [

Blue Ridge Mtns

Hot Springs
TN NC

Lovers Leap

Walnut Mtn [

French Broad River

I-40
Standing Indian
Hostel

Max Patch

Ground Creek [

Someone is Sleeping In My Bed

May 26, Hot Springs, NC

So much has happened since that night at Tri Corner. The trip down out of the Smokies was peaceful. It was nice to get down to the lower elevations, and see the rhododendron and mountain laurel in bloom. We had a long, downhill day, crossing the Pigeon River and I-40. Very strange to cross an interstate. We made our way up to Standing Indian hostel.

Well, that was quite an experience. The cabin we rented was quite cute, and we were feeling pretty good about things. We went to buy dinner (multiple burgers and a pork sandwich), take a nice shower, and eat. We met the conductor/train engineer,

the salesman of lightweight
towels, and Rocket, who was
supposedly in charge.

But when we got back to our beds,
people were sleeping in them.
Rocket did not want to be
bothered and said to work it out.
So I moved to the bunk house,
loosing my glasses and toothbrush
in the process. And then, the next
day, we found out that the
"laundry" was a wash board, and
most of the supplies were
outdated. Well, we were glad to
get out of there. But it was
certainly an interesting collection
of guests.

Seductive Trail

May 26, Hot Springs, NC

***

The next day, we climbed up to Groundhog Creek shelter. We had a wonderful evening there, cooking, eating, and sharing what I got from the English kid. Everyone was grateful, and the hikers from MI brought out more to share. We had a nice fire and totally enjoyed the evening, with Rainbow presiding.

The next day we hiked up to Max Patch. The weather was perfect. When we got up there, all of the shelter occupants were there, sunning and eating on the grass, taking in the spectacular views. Many A.T. Moments on that wonderful afternoon in that wonderful spot.

I've been told that the classic film, "Sound of Music", was filmed on Max Patch. Guess what song remained in my brain for so many days afterward. Do, Re, Mi.

Max Patch is a stunningly beautiful place. That gorgeous afternoon up there is burned into my brain, and maybe my soul; the warm sun, green grass speckled with wild flowers, and the 360 degree views.

There is something intense about being able to absorb the vibes from every direction all at once. Those mountains that we walked across, and that we would walk across in the days ahead shouted softly to us. We all shared the trees, grass, flowers, and air, all at once, and all together.

Beautiful views. Beautiful mountains. Beautiful Trail.

Beautiful. According to the dictionary, "physically attractive". Well, that sure seems to fit. We are drawn to beauty, attracted to it, and it is physical.

Sound familiar? Sounds a lot like sexual attraction to me. And it feels that way, too. It's very primal.

The attraction to the trail is strong enough to generate jealousy. Just ask the partner of someone who has been smitten by the trail.

Hot Springs

May 26, Hot Springs, NC

Been meaning to write for several days, but it's been, well, busy. We just spent a full zero mile day here, and you would think that would be plenty of time. It certainly was relaxing. We sat on the outdoor porch by the river, eating a fabulous salad, pulled pork sandwich, and drinking Angry Orchard hard cider. It was a hot day, but we were cool.

This is a friendly town, surrounded by the mountains and 2 rivers - very peaceful and beautiful. As usual, the laundry and shopping seemed to take more time than you would think. I had to get my new backpack belt installed. That took some playing around to get it right. Tonight, we went to the Iron

Horse for pork ribs, sweet potato puree, and cajun corn. There was live music - Celtic, but mountain music, fiddle and guitar. I love this town.

It was quite a challenge to get in here before 4, when the post office closed for the Memorial Day weekend. We did 2 consecutive 14 mile days. And since my pack was riding mostly on my shoulders, it was a quad vitamin I day, but we did it.

Tomorrow we head up again. I'll sure miss this town.

May 27, Hot Springs, NC

Well, a down day for sure. Last night, I had a terrible bout of diarrhea and vomiting. At one point, I went unconscious. I fell onto the floor on my side, and hit my head on the wall. I guess everything is ok, though, more or less.

I signed up for another night at the Alpine Motel here. I took some diarrhea medicine, and that finally stopped it. I was able to eat a lunch of a chicken sandwich, and just had a dinner of a pint of ice cream, since the diner is closed. I'm feeling weak and tired, but at least the diarrhea has stopped.

Not sure if I'll be strong enough tomorrow to hit the trail. It is 2000 feet of climbing, with temps in the 90's and possible afternoon thunder showers. The shelter is 11 miles away. The uncertainties are the biggest thing. I wish I felt better. Maybe tomorrow I will. Will See.

May 31, Flint Mountain Shelter, NC

***

Four days ago, we left Hot Springs. We met Rainbow, who was camped down by the river. I gave him my sewing kit, and some of what I got from the English hiker. After all, he had literally saved my butt when I ran out of toilet paper and he gave me his wipes. I'm not sure if I'll see him again. His feet are still bad. I'll miss him.

Well, what a difference a day makes. Feeling wonderfully healthy one day, and the next, plagued by agonizing physical distress. Quite a contrast.

But that is the trail, too. Hot and cold, wet and dry, clouds and sun, wind and calm, healthy and sick. Curiously, the good times help you get through the bad times, but the bad times rarely spoil the good times. Selective memory? Maybe.

Never under estimate the importance of toilet paper on the A.T., and share what you have. This happened over and over on the trail, sharing vitamin I (ibuprofen), batteries, water, food, duct tape, helping each other out, taking care of one another.

Rainbow was one of the most generous. He was a participant in the "rainbow gatherings", where money is not allowed. When you are up in the mountains on the trail, there is no place to spend money, so it is quite useless anyway.

Caveman said his family feared that he would have to face "highwaymen" on the A.T. We both laughed about this.

"This is a stick up. Hand over all of your oatmeal."

In 40 years of hiking the A.T., I never once witnessed anyone getting robbed of anything. That's just not how the trail works.

Caveman said that he never was worried about being robbed, but that he felt most vulnerable when trying to cross a highway. The speed with which cars move became inconceivable to us. We were adapted to a different time scale. Things don't move that fast in the natural world. Now it is easier for me to understand why there is so much road kill on the highways. We did not want to become road kill.

Rainbow was always smartly attired in a very functional duct tape inspired wardrobe. Duct tape. A hiker from GA told me they call it "Alabama Chrome". I don't know what they call it in Alabama. But whatever you call it, we all rely on it from time to time.

Oh, and the sewing kit? I did not think I would need it to fix the new backpack belt I picked up in Hot Springs. Little did I know.

Other People's Sweat

May 31, Flint Mountain Shelter, NC

There are 5 of us here in the shelter tonight: the father/daughter couple from Indiana, Princes, the teacher from TN, and Caveman and I. The kids, all 4 of them are tenting nearby. They are cute, to-be doctors and lawyers, just graduated, ready to start grad school, out for a few days, enjoying themselves.

Four days ago, we left Hot Springs. There were great views of Hot Springs from Lover's Leap. I was glad that I was feeling ok, and that the climb was going ok after being sick. That night, I ate a whole huge dinner. It was good to be hungry again. And the views from the fire tower were fabulous. All of the Smokies from Mt

Cammerer on down.

The next day was a tough day, with lot's of climbing, hot and muggy, and rain. Finally, the rain stopped and the sun came out. I began to relax, and stretched out on a nice, big cool flat rock by the trail. I fell asleep, a peaceful, sound sleep.

Suddenly, I woke up to the sound of thunder, and the sky was dark. I quickly got going. Soon it started to rain again. By the time I got to the shelter, I was wet, but not soaked.

Yesterday, we hiked from Laurel Mountain Shelter to Jerry Cabin Shelter, right over the ridge. It was unexpectedly awesome. We were totally unprepared for the spectacular views. It was hard climbing up on the rocks, but the narrow ridge afforded incredible views in both directions simultaneously: TN on the left, NC on the right. And it was cool and sunny at the same time.

It started to rain right after we got in here. It was a short day for us, down from Jerry Cabin Shelter, only 5.9 miles. We went over Big Butt and got a fabulous view of the farms in KY, all the way to the Cumberland Plateau, very beautiful.

Then we descended, and passed the small cemetery up on the mountain. There were 3 headstones. Two were soldiers from NC that joined the Union during the civil war. They were coming to a remote cabin up there to rendezvous with their families, but rebel troops found them and killed them, along with the 13 year old boy who was a lookout for them. It was sobering to be in that clearing, with the mowed grass around the tombstones, right there on the A.T. The civil war was not very far away from here, and it is very complicated. The mountain people were, and are, very independent, and did not in general support the rebel cause. They did not believe it was right to earn a living off of other people's sweat.

Coming upon that cemetery high up on the mountain moved me tremendously. I could not get the image of what had happened there out of my mind: how those mountain people died rather than fight on the side that would subjugate people. They sure knew something about freedom, and I was beginning to learn how much I did not know about the South.

Freedom. Paradoxically, there is a lot of freedom in the South. I have vivid memories of that ride back to the trail in GA, riding with my hiking buddies in the back of a pickup truck, our hair blowing in the wind, cruising among the folds of those beloved mountains. And we had the freedom to just stop and camp almost anywhere (outside of Smoky Mountains National Park). Freedom.

But then, slavery, too. But not around here.

Wind

June 2, Bald Mountain Shelter, NC

What a difference a day makes!
So much nicer today than
yesterday. It started out with
promise. The sun was trying to
poke through. I got an early start
by trying to find the privy (after
going down the wrong trail), and
then getting 5 liters of water for
the group down the interminably
long trail. It was very cold, but
after coffee and oatmeal, it felt
good to get walking.

The hike was uneventful, with a
short stop at the highway to
dispose of trash and help
Wondering Snail with a phone
call. But Big Bald was
spectacular! Could not stay up
there long because of the cold
and the wind, but incredible
views. And the shelter here is

nice, with only 2 local kids sharing it with us. Wondering Sparrow is tenting nearby.

But yesterday was horrendous! It started to rain almost as soon as we got up. Of course, we were reluctant to begin hiking in it, but it was fairly light and warm, so it really was not bad. I even managed to have lunch with the sun beginning to come out.

But by the time I got to the top of the ridge, I noticed a dark cloud approaching, and then the sky opened up! It poured, and the wind howled, and trees began to blow over. In two minutes, I was completely soaked. Only one thing to do - hike. And hike! Through the deluge of water on the trail, as the trees continued to topple over. One 4" diameter dead tree would have hit my pack if I had not jumped.

It got worse. Like an apparition, two young hikers appeared and disappeared in the torrential fog. Neither knew where the shelter was.

I hiked. I was getting cold and scared. I kept moving. Another hiker appeared and disappeared.

Finally, there was the sign. I was never so grateful to see a shelter. It was jammed. I changed into dry clothes under the overhang outside, and got into my sleeping bag, fingers numb, shivering. As we slowly warmed up, Wondering Snail told stories of ghosts in the Chattahoochee Forest.

A memorable evening after a memorable day. But that's the A.T., too.

It certainly is possible to get lost on the A.T.,

especially in conditions of blowing rain and fog. The trail is marked by white blazes painted on the trees, rocks, or posts, 2 inches wide by 6 inches tall. If the trail makes a sudden turn ahead, there will usually be 2 blazes, one above the other, with the top one offset slightly in the direction the trail will turn. Side trails and trails to shelters that intersect with the A.T. are usually blazed in blue. On that windy, stormy day, I was concerned that I walked right by the side trail to the shelter. This would not have been good, in those conditions.

I carried a long distance hiking book that contained tabular data recording shelter locations, water sources, and road locations. I almost always was equipped with typographic maps that would be of enormous help if I ever lost the trail. If you don't see a white blaze in awhile, say 1/4 mile, turn around and retrace your steps until you see the blazes again. As a last resort, rely on your typographic map and compass. People do get lost. Inchworm, a thru hiker from TN got lost in Maine in 2013, and died 2 miles from the trail.

Wondering Snail was a Hare Krishna, and an interesting hiker. He was limited to about 3 miles/day because of a medical condition. So he went slowly but deeply in his flowing robe. His ghost stories seemed real to us that night, as the wind howled.

Trees fall in the woods all the time. If you spend any time in the woods, you probably have heard them fall, sometimes on a sunny, windless day. That is one thing.

But when many trees start falling, all around you, that is another thing. It was probably the scariest day on the trail yet.

You have to look up.

Magical, Mystical A.T.

June 4, Uncle Johnny's Hostel,
Erwin, TN

Finally, we are here, and it sure feels good.

The trip down to No Business Shelter was uneventful. The trail and shelters now are maintained by the TN Eastman Hiking Club, instead of the Carolina Hiking Club. It seems they are simpler: no Privy, no bear cables, and a cement block shelter! Who knew.

On the way down from No Business Shelter this morning, my backpack finally fell apart and came flying off, grazing my leg. But instead of worrying about it, I just figured that I would figure out what to do when the time came.

We got down into town easier than expected. Caveman said it was like an airplane coming in for a landing. Each switchback is like circling. More and more of Erwin was revealed at each sweep.

We took wonderful showers and took the shuttle to the wrong end of town, but that let us eat our way across town.

We got to the shoe repair shop. There was a huge model railroad setup consuming half the shop, and all kinds of saddles and riding gear and boots, not to mention shoes. The guy does all sorts of work, and he said he could fix my shoulder straps. Oh joy, maybe I can still use my backpack!

As we moved to McDonalds, a woman asked if we needed a ride. She picked us up, along with a bunch of hikers, and brought us to Aztec, so we could gorge on Mexican food, and where the shuttle could get us back to the hostel.

I will remember the ride back for a long time. The music was wonderful Reggae. The mountains where sheathed in a purple/gray cloud bank. I looked up into those beautiful mountains that we had just walked across. I was in tears. An A.T. moment.

But the biggest surprise of the evening was seeing Indian Brave popping out of the van that came to get us. And then I got a text from Test Run about setting up a reunion on Roan Mountain soon, so we all might be together again! Wow, how can the A.T. do this?

Well, I think it has to do with dimensionality. There are so

many dimensions to the A.T. The
beauty, the pain, the joy, the
suffering. But in one sense, there
is only one dimension - miles. So
all the players can move around
on the trail, but they always pop
up someplace, but who knows
where? The magical part. The
mystical part. The mountains. The
A.T.

June 6, Curly Maple Shelter, TN

Erwin was great. Yesterday I
walked up the hill 1 1/2 miles to
go to Engle's Cafe. I'm glad I
did. It was a local place, and
they were very nice. The owner's
daughter did pencil sketches of
some of the old burial sites on
the mountains. I told him about
the ones I had seen. It was a
good connection.

I like Erwin. It certainly is the

most Christian town I have ever been in, and I would say that most people seem to be living by those values. It feels that way. The ten commandments are everywhere.

Last night, I sat down and figured out the milage and days all the way to Damascus. It's only a little more than 2 weeks. I'm very excited about that, and now I think I can make it. It certainly seems possible now. And, according to a southbound hiker, it looks like we will see the rhododendrons blooming. And we have the reunion Monday. A lot to look forward to.

It seemed that the trail today was easy. Got to the shelter much faster than expected.

All going well.

It is magical. One hundred miles of trail was magically searched for so many of our hiking acquaintances, all going different speeds, hours/day hiking, days to resupply, and depositing us all here to connect and enjoy each others company one more time.

Magical, yes. But you do need a backpack, a rather prosaic requirement, and mine had been coming apart for years. I have used the same antique external frame backpack for 45 years or so, and have gotten quite used to it. I can retrieve things in the dark.

But things do break down with age. So I had parts shipped into Hot Springs and later, Glasgow. And I had the leather work done in Erwin. Completely obstinate.

There is a saying on the A.T., "Hike your own hike". Do your own thing. Do it your way. So you see all sorts of strange ways out there. One time, when a hiker saw my pack, he picked up his phone and said a call was coming in from the Smithsonian Institution. They were interested in my backpack.

But I still use it.

Are We Changing?

June 6, Curly Maple Shelter, TN

Are we changing? Caveman said he thought he was changing, but was not sure how. He asked if I thought I was changing. I thought about that.

Well, physically, I sure have changed. The scale at Uncle Johnny's said I weigh 153. I'm doubting that, but I sure am thinner, maybe even skinny. But I feel good, and go up the hills easily.

But how else am I changing? I do think I'm more emotional now. The ride back on the shuttle, with my eyes tearing up when I saw the mountains, was certainly different. I could not even describe it to Jose when I spoke with him later.

I am very relaxed, and confident.
I feel good about being able to
handle whatever comes up. And it
should get easier.

I'm very comfortable living in the
woods. It has become routine. One
of the thru hikers said that a
friend of his wanted to sleep in
his hammock when he got home.
His wife was not amused.

But I think it is the depth of the
emotions I feel that is different.
I really, really feel now.

And I now avoid stepping on any
living thing as I walk along, even
an ant. I seem to have a new
respect for the life around me.
Being immersed constantly in the
depths of all this nature is
intoxicating. It has changed me. I
don't know if it is permanent. But
it is powerful.

And another change. The senses are definitely enhanced. Take smell, for example. I could usually smell a bear before I could see it. And the smell of a fire, or even just the charcoal from a previous one, travels far. And a privy? I can smell that literally a mile away.

I believe some of the enhanced sense of smell has become permanent. Some of it is probably training.

Nothing like the A.T. to sharpen your senses.

Sky

June 10, Over Mountain Shelter,
TN

This is a beautiful shelter, maybe
one of the best. It is an old barn
on a gravel road, not far off the
A.T. The barn is at the head of a
valley that looks out to fields
and an orchard, framed by
mountains on both sides.

Donut made a fire and cooked a
blueberry muffin in tin foil on
the fire. He really likes to cook.
He brought up a head of broccoli
to add to his couscous.

It's our last night out before
resupply, so I used up the last of
everything. Two Ramens, some
freeze dried hamburg and corn.
It was, of course, delicious.

Tomorrow, we will head to the

Mountain Harbor B & B for our
reunion with Test Run and
Slaughter. I've been looking
forward to that for quite some
time. It will be nice to see them
again.

The walk down there might be
uncomfortable. It is drizzling
now, and they are predicting rain
for the next 3 days. It's 9 miles,
with a 700' climb, but then a 2500'
descent, probably in the rain.
Hopefully it won't rain all day,
but at least we can dry out at the
B & B.

It's a little strange here in the
loft of the barn. It's huge. There
are 3 or 4 groups of sleeping
bags, with 4 or 5 people in each
group. The groups seem to be
fairly independent, not like in a
shelter, where it is mostly one big
group.

The last couple of days before today have been wonderful for hiking, sunny, dry, and cool. Friday was a tough day, 12.8 miles, and a lot of climbing. Beauty Spot Bald was indeed beautiful, as so many of the balds are. It's too bad that hikers, particularly women, are being harassed by motorists that can drive up there.

Then it was time to head over Unaka Mountain. It's over 5000', so that was quite a climb to do at the end of the day. But the rocks are some of the oldest in the world. They have crystals and are very dense, and often perfectly cubical. The top of the mountain is covered in hemlock and red spruce. It looks like Vermont. But it was a horrendous descent, so I was real glad to get into Cherry Gap Shelter.

The trip up to Roan Mountain was a tough climb, but ok. The shelter up there is the highest on the A.T., at 6275'. The shelter is an old wardens cabin, so I was glad it was enclosed. Before it got too cold, we had a conversation with Blistas and Sherlock, who agreed with me that the big bang theory is bunk. That seemed to surprise everyone, but Blistas agreed with me that expecting the universe to have an edge was like thinking the earth is flat. We could have gone on longer, but it was too cold. So we all slept on the floor, and I woke up when a group of 3 from Atlanta came in after dark.

The hike across the Roan Highlands was interesting, especially the balds, which were covered in blooming rodys and flame azalea. We met a lot of day hiker civilians, and they all stopped to ask us questions. They gave us delicious chocolate truffles and some candy bars. Trail angels.

So just now, guess who just showed up. Indian Brave. He did a 15 mile day to get here. He really wants to be at the reunion. And guess what? According to Delta Force, Candy Cane is 2 days ahead of us. Don't know how, but he is. Small world, this trail is.

You never know what the conversation will turn to around the campfire. Everything pointed to the sky for us during those days. We were up high, and we felt it. The balds were grass, flowers, and sky. And in the stunted trees, a lot of sky. So our thoughts that cold, starry night around a campfire high up on a tall mountain turned celestial.

Until it got too cold.

Breakfast

June 12, Mountain Harbor B&B,
Roan Mountain, TN

I'm sitting on the porch, enjoying
a bit of solitude. The breakfast
here this morning was fabulous,
far better even than I could have
imagined. Smoked salmon and
herbed cream cheese muffins.
Pancakes with walnuts and honey.
Fresh melon and pineapple. Three
kinds of eggs, one of them with
pirogies. Ham. And so many other
things. Fabulous!

But the loft in the barn? Chaos.
Maybe 15 hikers trying to use one
plugged up bathroom/shower. And
hotter than hell last night. But
still, I slept well.

The walk down yesterday was not
easy. Only 9 miles, and most of it
down hill. We needed to cross

two mountains, Hump and Small
Hump, but they were not small at
all. They are bald mountains.
Normally, balds are fun, but it
was a blowing, cold rain, blowing
very hard. I had trouble standing
up. Caveman said that as he
looked through the fog, he could
barely make me out, struggling
slowly up against the wind, with
my poncho out horizontally. Well,
I sure was glad to get back down
in the trees.

Last night, we had a very nice
visit with Test Run and the
Applewoods (Zen and #5) and
Indian Brave. A lot of trail news
about what's up there in VA and
about hikers we know - trail
gossip. Looking forward to
another night of visiting, and of
course another breakfast.

You can't imagine how important food becomes.
We all crave and hallucinate food. And to have

that satisfied in such an overwhelming way is ...
bliss.

Cool Water

June 14, Moreland Gap Shelter, TN

Well, not my favorite day. In fact, in terms of the terrain we were hiking across, my least favorite since Springer. Not difficult - little climbing. But it just kept going in circles. Down low, choked with rhododendrons. Lung congesting pollen. Lots of water that we were advised not to drink because it drained from farmland. And did I mention the mud? Or the mosquitoes? Or the lack of a breeze on a humid day?

There were a couple of nice moments. The cascade, where I chilled my feet for awhile. And the view, not too distant, of the town of Roan Mountain, I think.

But yesterday was wonderful. It

started with another fantastic breakfast at Mountain Harbor. Four Star. Unbelievable.

After crossing some abandoned fields, and traversing a bald with wonderful views, we headed down to Jones Falls. They were gorgeous! I took off my shirt and climbed to the rocks nearer the top, and cooled off in the spray. Then the trail went down to the Elk River, and followed it for awhile. It was nice being in some new, different terrain.

Mountaineer Falls Shelter is a nice one, with a third floor penthouse that Caveman enjoyed. There were two cute young kids from Michigan, and then a 67 year old marathon runner hiker who was doing 20 mile days. He had to stop when he had blood in his urine.

I don't understand pushing so hard that you break yourself. I asked him how you know when you've gone too far. He said you know it when it is too late. Of course, if that happened to me, I would have to get off the trail. It would be the end of my adventure, to be avoided at all costs.

June 15, Laurel Fork Shelter, TN

What a beautiful spot this is! We are up on a narrow ridge, overlooking the Laurel River. It is like a guard tower up here. You can see anyone approaching on the trail. The shelter is of native stone. It faces the gorge, and you can hear the river. There is a cut through the rock in back that used to have a logging railroad in it. Opposite the river, one of the steepest mountains I have ever seen rises up, at maybe a 70 degree angle. It is wooded, and I don't know how those trees hang on up there.

The walk today was a good one. We climbed up on the ridge, free of the rhododendrons at last. Then we descended to Dennis Cove Road, to the Black Bear resort. We ate lunch and resupplied.

Then it was descending down the stone steps, and through the railroad cut to Laurel Falls. I got into the pond in front. Quite cold.

Then up to this shelter. A beautiful day hiking.

June 20, The Place Hostel, Damascus, VA

Yesterday, that's all we could think about: getting to Damascus. After all, if you can make it to Damascus, you can make it all the way. Will see.

We were exhausted. Out of trail food, down to peanut butter and some stale flat bread that was stuck together. It was hot, and we were tired, after two consecutive 16 mile days. So we were rushing, not enjoying it at all.

And then, finally, I said "So What?". I slowed down. I crossed the border into VA, elated.

Water. We had been fighting against it for a couple of months. But now, it was getting hot, and water was our friend.

Rivers. Waterfalls. Watauga lake. Cool, cleansing, welcoming water.

But we were eager to get to VA., too. And you won't get there if you don't walk. We were hikers, after all, and our occupation was to walk. I had people ask if I did much fishing along the trail. This section, with plenty of flowing water, would have been a good section to do that. But it almost really was like we had a job to do. Our primary goal was to walk. There was always the tension between having a nice, relaxing walk, and doing miles. We looked at the maps to determine a reasonable destination for the next re-supply, and had to make sure we had enough food to actually get there, along with a little extra for safety. Sometimes, if there was not a lot of climbing on the trail ahead, we became greedy for miles. Two consecutive, 16 mile days was probably too much for us. But we did it! Damascus, and VA, beckoned.

Map 4 - VA

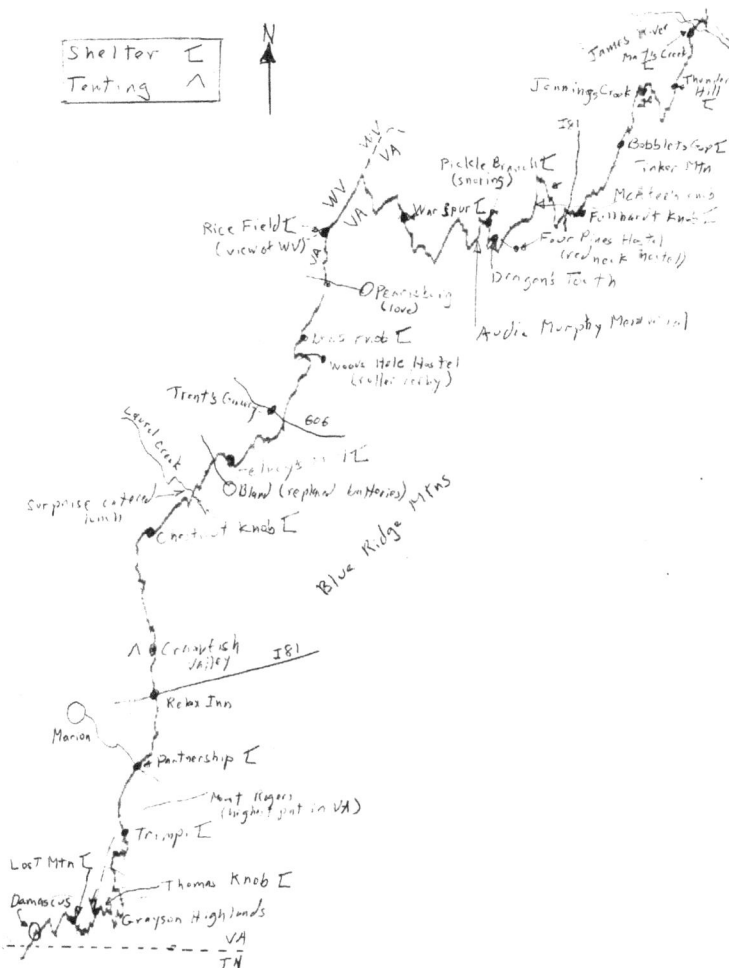

Shelter ⌐
Tenting ∧

N

James River
Ma 7's Creek
Jennings Creek
Thunder
Hill ⌐

Pickle Branch ⌐
(snoring)

I81

Bobbletts Gap ⌐
Tinker Mtn

McAfee's Knob
Fullhardt Knob ⌐

Rice Field ⌐
(view of WV)

War Spur ⌐

Four Pines Hotel
(red neck hotel)

Dragon's Teeth

Open ridge
(love)

Bass knob ⌐

Audie Murphy Memorial

Woods Hole Hostel
(roller derby)

Trent's Grocery

606

Helvey's ⌐

Laurel Creek

Bland (replace batteries)

Surprise catered
lunch

Blue Ridge Mtns

Chestnut Knob ⌐

Crawfish
Valley

I81

Kebo Inn

Marion

Partnership ⌐

Mnt Rogers
(highest pnt in VA)

Trimpi ⌐

LocT Mtn ⌐

Thomas Knob ⌐

Damascus

Grayson Highlands

VA
TN

Damascus

June 20, The Place Hostel,
Damascus, VA

Finally, Damascus! After so long
looking forward to it, and we're
here now.

Yesterday I crossed the border
into VA, elated. I spotted the blue
side trail to the spring. The water
I got at the last shelter tasted
terrible. So I went down and
filled up. It was cold and
delicious. Then I found 2 salami
sticks and the last of my cheese,
so I had a little lunch.

Then a young blond kid showed
up - Provisions, I think he called
himself. We talked about blood
lines, northern people, bears,
peanut butter, embalming, the
planet ... For maybe 45 minutes.
Then I calmly headed into town.

I took the creeper trail to the hostel, and had a nice shower. Then I went to the dairy place and had a burger, fries, and milkshake.

The Place hostel was nice. Very quiet. Just me, Caveman, and Bee Man last night.

Today, a lot more people showed up, but this house is so big and airy, no problem. We had blueberry pancakes at Cowboys, burgers at the diary place, and BBQ. We got an unrequested ride from a generous local woman right to the hostel when we were loaded down with groceries.

Last night, I finally got around to doing the numbers. Turns out I can't expect to get to CT unless I average 14 miles per day, to get there by the end of September. But if I give myself an extra week or two into October, I can do it with around 12.5 miles/day. To me, that seems much more manageable. And to hike in NY and CT in October would be fantastic! What a way to finish! Now I can rest easier.

Damascus, VA is an iconic A.T. town. It is one of the few towns that the trail goes right through, so long distance hikers don't have to do road walking or hitch-hiking to rest and resupply.

And something else. Trail lore has it that if you can make it to Damascus, you can make it all the way to Maine. North of Damascus, the mountains are not generally as tall, and the trail not as steep, as what we had been through, at least until you get to New England. So we all greatly look forward to Damascus.

Damascus hosts the annual "Trail Days" celebration, a large hiker reunion party. And then there is the Creeper Trail, a bike and hiking trail that the A.T. shares for awhile. It is built on the abandoned bed of a rail line that had been used for hauling timber out of the mountains. Damascus is a great town with an economy based on eco-tourism.

"The Place" hostel exemplified the values of this trail town. No charge to stay in a large house with bunk beds and showers, contributions welcomed. Nothing is locked up. Just like the trail. The whole town is in an A.T. frame of mind.

Feral People

June 23, Thomas Knob Shelter, VA

I'm sitting here in this beautiful place, with the wild ponies. Wild. It sure is nice to see wild ponies. Manilla told us this story about a wild young man trying to ride a wild pony. I guess that's what we are now - wild. Feral people. We are living in the wild. And I guess that is why it feels so good.

We need to be wild. To let out all of the stuff that civilization has suppressed, like our connection to nature - to the planet. To the trees and mountains and animals. To all of the things that we have lost our connection to.

It was tough getting up here from Lost Mountain. Two thousand foot climb, and 13 miles, but not nearly as bad as I would have thought. Feels good to have done that.

Yesterday was fun. An easy 6 mile hike, including part of the Creeper Trail. I soaked my feet in the water under the bridge.

The day before was the solstice, so I fulfilled my nudity by skinny dipping under the bridge while the cyclists rode overhead.

June 24, Grayson Highlands State Park, VA

I'm sitting on top of a rock outcrop. I can see miles in almost every direction. The wind is blowing across here. The fog has just lifted from the lowlands, and I can see blue sky above. And I'm feeling good - very good.

I've hiked maybe 1/2 mile from Thomas Knob Shelter. It's a mixture of open pasture, black berries, and stunted trees. Very, very beautiful, and I'm feeling very connected to it.

I've been thinking a lot about this notion of wild. How we have become, and are becoming more wild. What exactly does that mean?

If feels like I belong here, in these mountains, on this planet, and it feels so good to belong. Of course we have evolved here, so we really are home. Being here for this period of time has given us time to connect with who we really are. How all of this is deep inside us. Because we have evolved here. We are home.

I have been struck from the very beginning of this hike how much being in these woods and meadows reminds me of being home. Of being a child again, free. No school to go to. Just enjoying the woods, hills, ponds. Being close to what I really am. What is inside of me. What I am really made of.

We had been on the trail 9 weeks, and were beginning to merge into the world we were in. We were connecting to it in a powerful way, and were very aware of that connection.

There is a scientific hypothesis, biophilia, that helps explain what I felt so deeply up there on the mountain. It says that we are attracted to living systems because we evolved in them. So there are reasons for those deep feelings. Just google "biophilia'.

In our culture, so many of us are isolated from the natural environment. I have come across people who would not be surprised if the sun rose in the west. Environmental illiteracy is more widespread than you might believe. Maybe that's why such destructive things are done. And the planet is burned, instead of books. Not malice, just ignorance. And greed. But not here. The trail teaches.

I remember that afternoon cool off under the bridge. Trail lore has it that you should hike naked on the solstice. Well, I did not do that. But I hung onto the bridge timbers, letting the swiftly moving water levitate my body and wash it clean, unencumbered by a thread of clothing.

But being clean meant losing the natural water repellent that builds up on your hair and skin. Water just beads up on the layer of dirt, sweat and oil. Your body naturally sheds a light rain. Feral people water repellent.

Loneliness

This is the first time I'm camping in a long time, and it's the first time on the hike that I'm camping alone.

I'm lonely. I just finished looking at the photos of home and Jose and Vida. I welled up with emotion. How I wish I could teleport up to that screened in porch.

But I'm here, and so are the bugs. Mosquitoes, flies, deer fly, and some bumble bees (the rhododendrons are still! blooming). I set up the tent, which was stuck together. I hung a bear rope, and hopefully it works.

When I got down here, I expected to see a spring and stream. That's what the book said. But instead, I found some puddles. The water seemed to be moving, and it was cold. It tastes pretty good.

I only did 6 miles today. I came from I-81 and the Relax Inn with Bee Man. We had a hell of a time finding where the trail starts on this side. We wound up missing a chunk, but hiked the road 3 times! No blazes, and old blazes that were wrong.

Anyway, when I got here, I was too tired, and it was too hot, to climb up 1000 feet of Mount Walker, then down to get to the river. I decided not to. That will make it easier for Caveman to catch up with me. But it's not easy, not being with Bee Man or Caveman. Hope that we pop into the same time frame later.

We had a ball at the Relax Inn

last night. Blistahs and the gang were in room 111, and they made rum drinks for us, and we listened to the musicians play and sing. It sure was good to be there.

Yesterday Bee Man and I stopped at the Settlers Museum. A nice demographic, geographic, and historical view of the area in these mountains and hills.

Like many, maybe most, long distance hikers, I enjoy solitude, and got plenty of it on the A.T. Caveman and I usually hiked independently, unless the weather was dangerous. But most of the time, we hiked alone. I relish the solitude.

Before that night at Crawfish Valley, I had not spent a single night alone. I was lonely.

Before I started the hike, I expected to have to deal with loneliness a lot. But I immediately became a member of a tribe. We lifted each other's spirits. Encouraged each other. Dispelled a lot of loneliness.

That night at the Relax Inn (with color TV, the sign in front said) sure lifted our spirits. We sang a song, "Wagon Wheel". It talks of a young man hitch hiking from cold New England to his girlfriend in the South. All of the geographical places mentioned in the song are places we were near. It talks of wind and rain, and southbound trains, so it became our theme song. Whenever I hear it, it always brings back vivid memories of those times on the trail.

Caveman and I had been hiking on and off with Bee Man since TN. He was the only hiker that I ever saw on the trail wearing knee socks. Born in England, he became the island bee keeper for Nevis, an island in the Caribbean, and the birth place of Alexander Hamilton, as he always reminded us. The connections he developed to the birds, bees, and people on the trail inspired us.

We enjoyed the time we spent together at the Partnership Shelter. The shelter has a hot water shower, and a toilet. And for 50 cents, you could take the bus into Marion. I still remember Bee Man hitching back with pizza for us. Only one piece was missing, for the guy that gave him the ride. And then there was his trick of layering on all of his wet clothes at the laundry to save money on the drier. It was hot, so it worked. We did have fun.

Storms

July 1, Chestnut Knob Shelter, VA

Wow, am I glad to be here. And I don't just mean here at this fabulous shelter. I mean on this beautiful planet. I mean glad to be alive!

That was an incredible storm this morning. I first heard the thunder far off in the distance, when I was coming over the small hill. I figured I would have time to get over it to the road. As it got closer, I put the cover on the pack, and the plastic bag on the sleeping bag. As soon as I was finished, it started to rain.

But then the wind started, and it sure did blow. I put my poncho on, and watched as the trees started bending. I looked up, over my steamed up glasses, and started dodging falling debris. The lightening was blasting the ridge. And then a big top, maybe 10 inches in diameter, dropped on the trail about 30 feet in front of me. I am glad to be alive!

After it calmed down, I slowly made my way up the mountain, 2000 feet. I looked for dead hikers in the tangle of downed trees near the road. On the way, we squeezed some water out of the spring that fed a pond. The last water, the sign said, for 12 miles. What a drag.

But the shelter is great. Stone, in the middle of the grass, at the top of the ridge.

July 3, Helveys Mill Shelter, VA

Well, the crapy weather continues. Yesterday was a very tough day.

After we went to bed up there on the ridge in Chestnut Knob Shelter, all hell broke loose. It blew, and the lightening sizzled and snapped. Tail Light and No Doubt were out there camping. They came running in. We had to tie the door down with Tail Light's hammock strap. And we could see a funnel cloud far off in the distance, illuminated in the flashes. I loaned clothes to No Doubt, since his were soaked.

The hiking was no better. Rocks everywhere, up and down. By mid day, my knees were so sore I could hardly move. I used my last prescription ibuprofen, but at the end of the day, Giggles gave me a whole bunch more. I was so grateful.

Today started so nicely. The first 5 miles of the hike was much better than yesterday. It was an old logging road - no rocks, roots, crap. Very few blow downs. I made good time to the creek, and no knee pain.

When I got there, a guy asked me if I was hungry. Silly question. He was the cook for the trail racers. They are world class runners, getting ready to compete at the World Games in Poland. They are averaging 40 miles/day! He offered me a bowl of pasta with meat sauce, which I appreciated very much. Then I hiked the rest of the way to the interstate near Bland.

Almost forgot. This morning, when I tried to sterilize my water, the machine would not work. Turns out the batteries were bad. Bummer! Blistahs let me use his to make 2 liters.

When I got to the road, a woman

named Glow came down. She was slack-packing the section, and her husband was picking her up. When I told her about my batteries, she offered to drive me into Bland to buy some. We had to go to a couple of stores, since batteries were in short supply because of the wide-spread power failures. But we got them, and then they delivered me to the trail head.

I wasn't on the trail long when I heard the thunder starting again. Oh no! I put the pack cover on, and the rain came down in buckets. I kept going up the trail until I was getting near the top of the ridge. The lightening was getting intense, so I dropped my poles and took off my pack. I positioned myself among some smaller trees.

Fortunately, the wind was not too

intense. Unfortunately, the lightning was. It blasted a tree on top of the ridge. I started wondering if I really wanted to keep doing this. I really don't want to die out here!

The lightening ebbed a bit, and I marched on. I got to the shelter, dried off, and ate. I'm snug in my sleeping bag now.

Well, other than the blue ball lightening I saw in the storm, that's just about it.

Of course, the scariest aspect of storms is the possibility of getting killed. As I recall, 5 people died in the mountains throughout the Southeast during those storms. Usually it was falling trees, and one was lightening.

Lightening. Awesome. Makes you feel small. Powerless. But strangely, calm. I'm sure some of that is getting used to it. Knowing what to do. But maybe some of that flows from the awe itself. Science is just now becoming aware of some of the benefits of awe. But hikers know.

Right around dusk that night at Crawfish Valley, a strange wind rose up quickly, with no thunder, lightening, or rain. It was my first experience with a derecho, which is a long-lived, straight-line wind storm. The one that hit me on June 29 resulted in 29 deaths and $2.9 billion of damage across the US. But I was in a protected, deep valley, surrounded by ridges. A little light debris came down on my tent.

Others were not so lucky. One woman at another location had a large branch punch right through her tent, with her asleep in it.

You learn to look up.

Other than getting killed, the storms provide excellent obstacles to your hike with the strategic placement of blowdowns. A blowdown is a tree, or sometimes a tangle of trees, down across the trail. You would think that it would be a simple matter to just walk around it, and sometimes this is true. But more often than not, the tree is on the side of the mountain, and the trail is embossed onto the side of the mountain. So you can't really go around it, but have to fight your way through the branches. Trying to get around one on a steep slope, my glasses were flung who knows where. Glad I had a backup pair.

Roller Derby and Paul Bunion

July 6, Woods Hole Hostel, near Pearisburg, VA

I thought I would never get here. For the first time on this hike, I got going on the trail the wrong way. I went up the side trail to the tower. Turns out it was a collection of 4 comm towers, with a lot of humming noise up there. So I went down, and headed onto the A.T. the wrong way. I did not notice it until I got to the viewpoint, around 1 1/2 miles away, and recognized that I had been there earlier. I had to turn around and go back, and the last part was all on rocks. So my "short" 6 1/2 mile day turned into a tough 10 mile day.

Cute place here, but the

proprietors are away, so I'll see it better tomorrow. I'm planning a 0 here tomorrow, to wait up for Caveman. Looking forward to the organic food.

Yesterday was a long, 15 mile day, including the re-supply at Trent's. I enjoyed a full pizza and chocolate shake. But resupply was a little dicey, unless you were looking for bear traps and the like. But I was able to get a couple of dinners, and a bunch of Little Debbie pies. They are pretty good.

Trent's is just a little corner of the country world, but they were certainly enjoying life. Made me think about how stressed we get in our regular lives, and for what?

The hiking was fairly easy, with very little elevation change.

There was a T-storm in the morning, but it was not a bad one, with not too much wind. And it cooled everything off nicely. I put on my poncho and just sat on a log until the lightening eased. Then I hiked on.

The rest of the day, it was a light rain that kept things cool. But it was a long hike to the shelter. When we got there, they had a good fire going, so we had a nice, congenial evening.

July 8, Doc's Knob Shelter, VA

Well, last night at Woods Hole was quite a shindig. The Konnarock crew of ATC trail maintainers was there, along with some neighbors. The crew was awesome. Two of the most tattooed young women said they did roller derby when they weren't maintaining trail.

They were tough. And the big, tall, dark young man from FL. And the Paul Bunion head of them. He likes to move rocks, his favorite thing, I understand.

Bee Man has gone with him to NYC. I hope his foot heals fast.

The food was fabulous, both last night, and breakfast. It was so nice to have real food for a change. I can't wait to have my free range poached eggs on fresh baked bread tomorrow.

I like this shelter, set in the rodys. But the water is poor. Should work, though. Two hot young firemen from Richmond came in here awhile ago. They were very nice, and gave me a snickers bar and some trail gorp.

I hope Caveman shows up here.

The A.T. was built, and is maintained by volunteers. The Konnarock crew does a lot of heavy lifting. They are dispatched to areas of the trail that need major work, including relocating and rebuilding. Members volunteer for a week of tough physical labor. There is no pay, but the Appalachian Trail Conservancy does feed them, no small task.

Caveman was spending some time with his family, so I decided I would take it real slow and easy, waiting for him to catch up after his visit. Bee Man decided he needed to "leap frog" part of the trail, going north. That would hopefully allow him time to get to Maine before his visa expired. So, for a bit, I would be hiking without my two hiking buddies. I missed them.

Love

July 11, Pearisburg, VA

Second 0 day here now. And I
sure do love those 0s. Finally,
Caveman caught up with me here.
The heat and blowdowns have
slowed him down as well. I'm
glad he is here now. I really
missed his company.

Though I have some mixed
feelings, I like this town. I'm
glad I'm here. The trip in was a
bit negative. When I popped out
of the woods and asked a woman
the way in to town, she rolled up
her window. Then she said she was
going the other way, but verified
that I could get into town by
going up the hill.

It was quite steep, along 4 lanes
of traffic, with a very narrow
shoulder. When I got to the top, I

looked down into town. It was quite dispiriting. Hardee's, DQ, the motels, gas stations. A highway town. A minimal sidewalk on one side, and no cross walks.

But then I got to the Plaza Motel, and signed up for 3 nights at $25/night. I figured Caveman could use a 0, and two 0s for me sounded appealing. After a shower, some Fanta, and all you can eat Chinese buffet, I felt a whole lot better. It was good to just veg out.

Then yesterday, I went to the post office. My box was there, and I mailed out the last of my cold clothes. I went to the hardware store and got my fuel refilled. The proprietor also publishes a small monthly paper. He asked me to contribute an article about what it was like out there during the storm. I would like to, but probably am too lazy. If I had email on my phone, I might be more inclined. Then I went next door, and bought a NOAA weather radio. I'm glad I have that.

After a mega burger lunch at Hardee's, Butterscotch spotted me. He was having a smoke in front of the Mexican restaurant across the street. He said it was Blistahs' 42 birthday, and for me to come on in.

Blistahs bought me a big margarita, and we had a great time listening to music and playing pool. He asked me what people thought about them on the trail. I asked, "You mean when you all wind up in a big pile in the shelter?" I said people were curious about the intimacies involved. He was glowing from the margaritas, and I think quite honest. He loves both Giggles and

Butterscotch. They are both really cute.

I completely understand what Blistahs is talking about with love. It is a deep, abiding love we have for one another out here. It is the kind of love and caring you don't usually see in the regular world. I have seen hikers sharing water when they don't know if they will have enough. That is the kind of selfless love I'm talking about. A deep, caring about one another. And in their three-some, it is even more intense.

It is that kind of trail caring that exists in Damascus, when "The Place" hostel can be completely unlocked, and no one is concerned. It is such a contrast with Pearisburg, where I heard people trying my door in the hopes of finding it unlocked and stealing something from me.

The contrast in towns is so vivid.
Damascus does not have any
chain stores or restaurants. But
here, it is almost all chains, and
they are bleeding this town dry,
siphoning off the wealth and
sending it away. A lot of people
are obese. It is difficult to walk
here. And the A.T. seems far, even
though it is only a mile away. I
keep wondering what it would be
like if a side trail from the A.T.
came right down to the old
center of town. Hikers would
come, and it could be the
beginning of a renascence for
this town. If only they knew!
Probably some do.

Like the lady running the motel
here. She washed my clothes, and
would not accept any money for
doing it. She says she does it for
all the hikers. And the women at

Rite Aid who took the time to find a single tube of travel toothpaste. She just got her power back this morning. Trail magic, even here, even now.

Being a slow hiker does have its advantages. I got to know so many hikers, and hike with them for a few days before they passed me. My first hiker family - Test Run, Slaughter, Zen and #5, and Indian Brave were now far ahead of me.

But there was another hiker family - Blistahs, Butterscotch, Giggles and Tail Light that Caveman and I got to know very well. They were faster than we were, but enjoyed spending more time in town than we did. So we kept up with them for hundreds of miles.

Giggles was probably the female hiker that I got to know best. I don't think I ever heard her complain about anything. She once said she thought woman do better on the trail than men. I think she is correct. I don't know if it is due to a little more body fat, better endurance, or more emotional resilience, or maybe all of the above. But the women I got to know certainly were proficient hikers.

We were delighted whenever we shared a shelter with Blistahs and the gang. They shared water, ibuprofen, batteries, rum, music, information and encouragement with us. Their generosity and enthusiasm flowed from the love they had for each other. We knew we would be ok when we were around them.

Because the trail goes within one mile of Pearisburg, it was a major re-supply point for us. A day hiker once asked us if we carried all of our supplies from GA. That is an interesting question. I did a quick calculation. I need at least 3 pounds of dried food per day, around 20 pounds per week. Since we had been on the tail for around 11 weeks, that would have required carrying 220 pounds of food starting out, just to get to Pearisburg. The question reveals a profound lack of understanding of our basic reality. We generally tried to limit our time on the trail between re-supplies to 6 days, which was an amount of weight we could carry somewhat comfortably.

Any town close to the trail with a supermarket was a good re-supply point for us. I bought plenty of oatmeal, pasta sides, tuna and fish in pouches, bagels, summer sausage (does not need refrigeration), and dried fruit like raisons. But some things were not available in the small sizes we needed, and then there were the niceties, like my Brazilian coffee, so I had them mailed to me in care of "general delivery", to post offices along the trail. The mail drops also usually contained the maps I would need for the next sections, and of course replacement clothes, boots, and equipment parts for my disintegrating backpack. I had been reluctant to rely on the postal service for things I absolutely needed, but I received all of my mail drops promptly.

The Big Picture

July 14, War Spur Shelter, VA

Raining. Again. I guess just about every day for a week or so. I was hearing thunder all day, but finally it caught up with me around 5 or so. Moderately heavy rain, not too much lightening, thank goodness. I pounded down the 1500 feet to the shelter, wearing just shorts. When I got in, the usual drill. Hanging wet shorts on a nail, stuffing wet socks up in the frame. No place for them. Empty out boots. There is a copper head under the shelter. Hope he does not come in.

But I had a real episode of trail moments today. It happened at Wind Rock. The sky cleared, and I looked out over the mountains in West Virginia. And of course, John Denver was in my brain.

Then it hit me. The trail is heading north now, almost completely. And the flat rocks look like at home. Yesterday, we saw the Allegheny Trail. It heads up to the Mason Dixon line. I'm heading north now, going home with every step, getting closer. I've been enjoying the south enormously, but soon, I'll be in the north. How strange! How wonderful!

And, of course, yesterday, walking over to West Virginia at sunset. It's sort of the north over there, and the 5th state.

It's good sometimes to see the big picture. We have been putting up with heat, humidity, very rocky trails, and it is getting old. But we are moving north, and I know we will get there.

And then there is the small picture. Coffee.

At home, I always enjoyed a nice cup of coffee around 3 pm. But on the trail, I usually didn't because it was just too much trouble to stop hiking, set up the stove, and boil water. But that afternoon, I had a terrible urge for coffee. I re-supplied in Pearisburg, so I had enough Brazilian coffee to brew for everyone in the shelter. We sipped our coffee, watching the sun set over West Virginia.

Oh. And that copper head snake? It poked its head out just below the dangling feet of a hiker sitting on the edge of the shelter floor. She noticed it, but did not even miss a beat in her conversation. No fear, at least not for her. And a big bonus. No mice in the shelter that night, for a change.

Mice. If you spend even a microsecond in a shelter at night, you will experience Mice. Hungry Mice. Persistent Mice. The very first time I hung my brand new pack in a shelter, mice drilled holes wherever I accidentally left trail goodies. Can't do that.

A very clever mouse inhibit device can be found in most shelters. A cord hanging from a rafter passes thru a hole in an upside-down tuna can. There is a little stick at the end of the cord, which is knotted below the can. That's where you hang your food bag. It usually works. But it is always fascinating watching the little acrobats swinging on the little trapezes.

We had been on the trail about 12 weeks. So, what exactly did we do in all that time? At its most basic, we were walking. Move the back foot to the front. Repeat. That's it.

But sometimes, you need to reverse course. One step forward, two steps back. Maybe you chose to go around a rock or tree on the wrong side, and have to back up. Sometimes, it's more serious. Perhaps you turned onto a side trail to get to a shelter. But the next morning, you can't remember which direction you came from. Could wind up back in GA if you don't watch out.

What is the trail surface like? There are some sections that are flat and smoothly paved. I remember a wheel chair accessible section in TN that we loved. Sometimes, you will have the pleasure of walking on soft pine needles, or sand, or gravel. Nice.

My favorite kind of trail goes over the bald

mountains. They have no trees, but are covered in grass, speckled in wild flowers. The trail is marked by posts painted with a white blaze. Usually there will be fantastic views, including the undulating trail, luring you onwards.

Sometimes, the trail crosses marsh land on beautiful boardwalks. Usually, though, it crosses these areas on simple log bridges, with 2 partially flattened logs or planks suspended above the mud on rocks or logs. Balancing on them as they shift around can be a little tricky. You dare not slip off, and get sucked into the swamp.

But most often, you will be walking on rocks. You use less energy if you step around them, rather than over them. All kinds of rocks. Metamorphic rocks with quartz and mica embedded in them. Volcanic rocks that look like they came from Mars. Perfectly flat rocks. Perfectly round rocks. Concave and convex rocks. Loose, rolling rocks that will try to twist your ankle. Wet, slippery rocks that will put you on your ass. Rocks that will rock back and forth as you step on them. Sloped slabs of ledge that will kill your knees after awhile. Pointed rocks that will stab your boots. Big boulders you need to climb over. So many rocks.

And then roots. Most of the trail is in the woods, where trees tend to grow. And because the soil is thin, they are right on the surface. And when they get wet, watch out. It's like walking on ice. And then, my favorite. Wet rocks and roots, combined. Cement it all together with mud. That way, when you slip off that wet root, you can land in the mud, and get your boot sucked off.

So much for flat trails. Since the A.T. goes through the mountains, you expect to be going up and down a lot. You would be right. If you hike all of it, you will need to climb half a million feet. That's like climbing Mount Everest 16 times!

When you are lucky, the trail is chiseled into the side of the mountain, and ascends at a reasonable rate. Even so, that will take your breath away. As it goes up, it changes direction in a switch back, doubling back on itself, but higher up. And this pattern is repeated, back and forth, up and up you go.

Sometimes the trail does not change in elevation that much. It clings to the side of the ridge, following it around the edge like the fluting on a pie crust. You cross a crease where you might find water. Then, as you get to the outside edge of the ridge, the trail suddenly makes a right angle turn as it follows the next ridge around. Round and round you go.

More likely, you will be ascending steeply. If it is your lucky day, there will be stone or wood steps. Or maybe it's a giant slab of polished granite that you have to crawl up. Try that when it's wet. The toughest for me is when you have to climb up cracks in a vertical ledge. The rock climbers love it. Not me.

You might think that down would be the opposite of up. Not true. Unlike up, down is easy on your lungs. But it is really hard on your muscles, and of course your knees. Got to go slow. Don't want to go tumbling down the mountain.

The feel of the walk changes over the course of the day. In the morning, when starting out, I was aware of a cacophony of pain. Blister on left foot, check. Right knee, I hear you. Left thigh, ok, I know you are still there.

But after a half hour or so, it quieted down, as the endorphins went to work. That's the sweet spot for me. A painless walk through the woods in the cool of the morning. I liked to walk for an hour and a half before I stopped for a break. It was disappointing when I had to waste the sweet spot on wet rocks and roots.

One of the joys of my life on the trail was my mid day nap. Hikers who knew me were not alarmed when they encountered me sprawled out on a nice, big, cool flat rock after lunch. I usually had a restful, 20 minute sleep. But a couple of times, I was rudely awakened by the rumble of thunder and the flash of lightening on the next ridge.

I love the late afternoon light in the woods, with the contrast between the deep shadows and bright, crimson orange sunlight, as the sun sinks lower. But walking at the end of the day was also the toughest, for me. Dog tired. Dragging. The shelter is almost always further than you thought it would be. And, of course, the pain comes back. But the relief when you finally take your pack off at the shelter, and take a deep drink of delicious water revives completely.

How wide is the trail? Usually, it is not wide enough for two hikers to pass without one pulling over. Maybe it's 16 inches wide. But hey, what the A.T. lacks in width, it makes up for in length, over 2000 miles.

What do you see when you are walking the A.T.?
Mostly, you see your boots. Usually, you need to
watch where you step, unless you are on smooth,
level trail, which is unusual.

And so, we walked. And walked. And walked.

Red Neck Hostel

July 19, Four Pines Hostel,
Catawba VA

I did not think I would like it
here, but I do. It's a 3 car garage
with some cots, sofas, old living
room furniture, and a good
shower and flush toilet.

And Joe. He is wonderful. 61
years old, and a railroad bridge
inspector. His truck has train
wheels to go on the tracks. I
would say this is the first red
neck hostel I have been in.

Joe is a very practical guy. He
gave us some good advice about
what to do if a bear approaches.
If he goes after your food, hit
him on the head with your stick.
And if he rears up, fight
aggressively. Ram your stick
down his throat. Won't find that

in any book. (Till now) And then there is the "red neck bridge" they built to get to the market while the highway bridge is out. He can drive his golf cart through there.

My knees sure need a rest. Dragon's Tooth yesterday was very tough. Lots of rocks, up and down, climbing on rebar, etc. They are very stiff and sore today. Sure hope they are better tomorrow, when we hit the trail again.

Lots of rain coming tomorrow, 70% probability in the afternoon, with more Saturday. But cooler weather is forecast, Low 80s instead of low 90s. Should be a lot better hiking weather.

And we could use the rain. We have been hiking across the mountain tops, without staying up there. The springs are all dry. But the streams are flowing down below.

I really wanted to write something about A.T. Moments a few days ago. We were crossing several roads in the vicinity of Sinking Creek. The trail crossed numerous pastures and hay fields. It was early morning, and still cool. As I looked down from a ridge, Caveman was crossing one as he peacefully floated on down below. And, as usual, I was overcome with bliss. I guess that's what A.T. Moments are - bliss.

If you have never encountered bears, Joe's advice might seem harsh. But we understand that if a bear figures out she can get your food, that is a problem bear. It can easily happen if someone who does not know leaves food on a picnic table to go to the bathroom. Once the bear associates the intense smells of the food with the smells coming out of your backpack, you are in trouble. And so is the bear. That bear likely will be put down by the rangers. And that is something hikers dread to hear.

Food. How do you make a hikers day? Food. So we all loaded onto the back of Joe's truck, and he delivered us to the local Homeplace Restaurant, and heaven. All you can eat, southern style cooking, and inexpensive. Fabulous.

And then, the next day, we were treated to fabulous pulled pork by one of our hostel mates, who bought food for all of us, and would not accept a penny. Turns out we had met him earlier, at the top of Roan Mountain, when he arrived with the group from Atlanta after dark. Small world, generous world.

The day before getting to Four Pines Hostel featured both solemn and humorous times.

The Audie Murphy Monument is just off the trail at the top of the ridge. Audie Murphy was the most decorated soldier of World War II, and he died in a plane crash near this site. A large pile of rocks left by visitors bears witness to the sacrifices made by so many soldiers. The messages written on or attached to the rocks salute comrades lost. Encountering that in such a quiet, remote place moved me far more than any

Memorial Day celebration I have ever experienced. So many of the hikers I encountered on my hike were Afghan or Iraq veterans, so I was connected to those messages in a way I never would have been before.

Shortly after leaving the monument, a very energetic hiker approached from the rear.

"You must be Will See", he guessed correctly. "Where are you headed, tonight"?

After he learned I intended to sleep at the next shelter, he asked, "Do you snore"?

Well, I was a bit taken aback. It seemed a bit personal for someone I just met. Then he explained that he was a serial thru hiker, doing many miles/day, and that he really needed his sleep. So if I was going to spend the night in the shelter, I better not snore.

I told him that I could not guarantee that I did not snore, but if I did, he could wake me up.

That night, I was awakened by loud snoring. His.

Stinky Water

July 24, Fullhardt Knob Shelter, VA

Sitting here, waiting for it to rain. It's thundering off in the distance. The forecast is for 70% chance of rain, with possible severe thunderstorms. We arrived here around noon. Trying to decide if we should stay. We had planned to go to the next shelter, but we don't want to deal with falling trees. Not sure we made the right decision.

There are 8 people here in the shelter now. They are section hikers from Ohio and Louisiana. They are heading south, and I think they might camp here.

The water here is from a cistern that originally served a cabin for the fire tower. The water is wet, but it stinks and looks like tea. I guess we will boil it.

The hike up here was only 5 miles. It was up around 1300 feet, but an easy trail. No rocks, just dirt, and easy grades with switchbacks. We are on the Blue Ridge now. It feels like GA again. I hope it continues this way. My knees are liking it.

The mountains on the other side were a real trip. Catawba has McAfee's Knob on it, and Tinker Mountain has Tinker's Ridge. During the revolutionary war, the folks who did not want to participate hid out there.

The rocks there are incredible. Silurian Sandstone from the Paleozoic, the brochure said. Huge blocks, lots cubical. Blocks thrown on top of each other forming caves and overhangs.

Tinker Mountain has cliffs with wonderful views. The cliffs were formed when Africa bumped into North America, a little while ago.

McAfee's is iconic, but seems smaller when you get up there than you would think.

I enjoyed those mountains, but sure hope the hiking will get easier on my knees.

July 27, Cornelius Creek Shelter, VA

Finally, just a "regular" evening in a "regular" shelter. The last few days have been intense, and not too much fun.

First there was the stinky water at Fullhardt. Then a very long, 14 mile slog to Boblets. The Blue Ridge Parkway was underwhelming. The trail was forced right up to the Blue Ridge Parkway or the rocks at the ridge top. The water at Boblets Gap Shelter was limited, not too nice water. And then, yesterday, 100 degrees with a heat index of 107! On my break, I got out Jose's picture and nearly cried. How I wanted to be home just then.

I got down to Jennings Creek, and just jumped in. Finally, enough water to get into. We made camp down there away from the creek a bit, and settled into our tents for the night. Good thing. Seems a lively party of local kids, complete with loud music, got underway.

We got up early and hiked up here. On the way up, I turned on the NOAA weather radio, and heard that a thunderstorm was just then pummeling Bastion, not far south. It had 1 inch hail, 60 mile per hour winds and continuous cloud to ground lightening. They were advising everyone to get indoors. Good advice, I'm sure. But...

So that got me to thinking about negative A.T. Moments. I guess I've been self censoring them, because I'm too exhausted by them to write. So bad, or no water, heat, humidity, aching knees, severe storms.

Hell, what would I do if that severe storm hit me? Hope that I got knocked unconscious by 1 inch hail? Or get struck by continuous lightening? Or maybe just wait to be hit by a falling tree?

Oh well. Time for bed.

Water. Can't live without it. Well, not for long.

So much of our day revolved around water. First thing in the morning, get the water for breakfast. Then, tank up, and make sure you will have enough to get to the next water. And so on, thru the day. I remember encountering a dry stream bed when I had just one sip left, and was counting on it. I made a small hole in the gravel, and cold water slowly flowed in. I was able to scoop out a liter in a few minutes, using my cup.

In the heat, and with a feral persons sense of smell, I picked up the aroma of Jennings Creek long before I could see or hear it. The sense of anticipation was great.

But it's not just water you need in the heat. I met a hiker who just flip-flopped from Maine. A flip-flop is a change in direction on the trail, usually necessitated by climate or calendar. The hiker from Maine was not heat acclimated, and he did not know about electrolytes. He was in bad shape. I hated the taste of the water after you dropped one of those pills into it, but I knew we needed it.

Teared Up

July 28, Thunder Hill Shelter, VA

It was a beautiful day to hike today. Cool and dry, sunny but not hot at all. We started out by catching the views at Black Rock.

Then I met an older couple. She spoke with a German accent, and had hiked the Smokies and the Alps. They were both interested in talking with me.

When I said that "trail moments" moved me to tears, I saw her tear up. She seemed embarrassed, but her husband saw it, and pointed it out. I think he better understood the intensity of what we were doing. He wants to hike because of her, I think, but now has a better sense of it all.

Then it was on to Orchard

Mountain. Hard to believe 250 people lived up here once. Now just one radar station in a beautiful meadow with fir trees. And great views!

On to the guillotine, an unstable-looking rock hanging above the trail. Met Happy Feet and Gaspur. Did not know it at the time, but the bridge over the James is named after Happy Feet. They came up to clean up the trail, and said their club alone put in 900 hours of work recently to fix storm damage. I thanked them.

Then on to here for a relaxed, long afternoon after only a 5.5 mile day. Tomorrow will be a 12.5 mile, fairly strenuous day to Matt's Creek.

Map 5 - VA, WV, MD

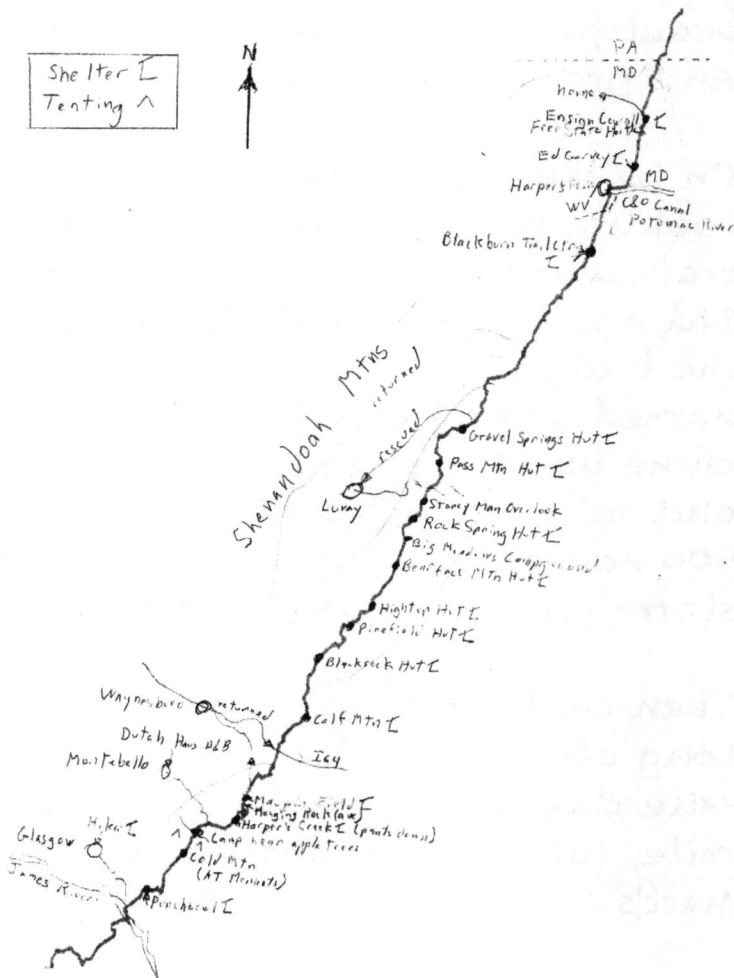

Shelter L
Tenting ∧

N

PA
MD

home

Ensign Cowall
Free State Hut
Ed Garvey
Harpers Ferry
WV
MD
C&O Canal
Potomac River

Blackburn Tr. Ctr

Shenandoah Mtns

returned

rescued

Gravel Springs Hut
Pass Mtn Hut

Luray

Stony Man Overlook
Rock Spring Hut
Big Meadows Campground
Bearfoot Mtn Hut

Hightop Hut
Pinefield Hut

Blackrock Hut

Waynesboro   returned

Dutch Haus B&B
Montebello

Calf Mtn

Icy

Maupin Field
Hanging Rock (air)
Harper's Creek (pants down)
Camp near apple trees

Glasgow
Hiker
Cold Mtn
(AT Meennots)

James River

Punchbowl

Shelter On 9th Street

July 31, Hikers Shelter, Glasgow, VA

Well, what a pleasant surprise! I'm sitting in the shelter on 9th street. It faces a grove of small maple trees. There is a fire pit with a grill, running water, and, would you believe, a hot shower.

It was hell to get here yesterday. No cell signal anywhere. We crossed the very impressive foot bridge over the James River, and tried to hitch for 20 minutes. No luck, so we started walking. Well, it was a winding, uphill death march in the sun and heat.

We got into town. The restaurant was closed because it was Monday, but we got sandwiches and sodas at the gas station. Finally, relief.

Then to the shelter. Caveman was imagining it filled with homeless people, but no one was there. We took showers (nice!) and relaxed. Then we got some dogs, chips, and VA wine and cooked dogs on the fire. I slept under the stars in the maple grove. Wonderful evening.

This morning, I had a restaurant breakfast. The proprietor is retiring, so it is the last day. Too bad.

This town has so much potential. Everything a hiker needs, all within easy walking distance. Too bad it is so hard to get here from the trail. I stopped by the town hall to thank them, and suggest the idea of a regular hiker shuttle. They seemed receptive.

I sure would like to see this town

prosper from eco-tourism. It seems to be a friendly, generous, quiet, pedestrian oriented town with mixed races. I hope they find their way to the future.

The James River bridge is a marvel. It is the longest pedestrian only bridge on the trail, and is built on piers from an old railroad bridge.

The trip into Glasgow was something we will remember, although we would rather forget. We were getting into a part of the trail where the resupply options were further off the trail. So we were looking at a 6 mile "death march", as Caveman put it. It was largely my fault, since I needed to pick up a package at the post office that contained parts for my still disintegrating back pack. But the shelter was a dream, and, the town too.

When Caveman was concerned about homeless people in the shelter, I asked him what his home address was, knowing full well that at that time, he did not really have one.

"So then there will be at least one homeless person at the shelter", I said.

Abstract Fears

August 3, on top of Cold
Mountain, VA

***

I can't help thinking about Larry.
He came into our shelter the other
day, not long before dark. He
announced that he did 20 miles,
and that he was a marathon
runner.

Fine, I thought. Just not my hike.
But then, he asked me what I do.
I really wanted to say that I eat,
sleep, and shit, but I thought that
would be rude. So I said that I
was a software engineer, and then
the moments disappeared, as he
forced more and more of the
other, abstract world onto me. I
hated it.

How is it that out here, we can

deal with truly life threatening situations, like running out of water, or being struck by lightening or a falling tree. These things really do happen. But for some reason, they seem to cause me less anxiety than a missed deadline (strange term, is it not?) would in the abstract world. I wonder how many of our fears are just abstract.

Larry's asking me what I "do" surprised me. On the trail, we learn about people inside-out. Their external characteristics like job, wealth, age, political affiliation and the like become invisible. But we see generosity, empathy, curiosity, creativity and courage clearly. They are from a person's core, but come to the surface on the trail. We see who they really are.

Abstract. The dictionary says, "existing in thought or as an idea, but not having a physical or concrete existence". Well, that pretty much describes a lot of what goes on in that other world. But not here. No question, for us, everything was real.

And so, our fears, also had become realistic. We knew that we had a very good chance of avoiding being struck by lightening by ditching our metal poles, and crouching near a medium sized tree away from the tallest trees. We knew that we could practically wring water out of a rock if we needed to. We understood bears, and were no longer afraid of them. We knew to look up when it was windy, and to move fast if need be. So, we felt safe.

But in that other world? That missed deadline? I can still remember the short breath, the bad taste in my mouth, and the anxiety. And yet, how bad could it possibly be? I guess I could loose my job. And then what? Become homeless? Well, I understood better now what that felt like. I could probably deal with it.

After spending time in the real world, we had learned what to expect, and there were not that many ways things could go. But the abstract world is much more complex. There is a lot more uncertainty. And a lot more anxiety.

That's why I so resented Larry's questions. I rather enjoyed being master of my world, and did not really want to be reminded of that other world, which was less predictable, less safe, and far less beautiful. At that moment, I strongly preferred the real world that I was in.

What Are A.T. Moments?

August 3, on top of Cold Mountain, VA

I'm sitting in the middle of a mowed mountain top. The grass is tall and brown, but there are tons of blue, purple, yellow and red wild flowers in it. I have a good 180 degree view of the mountains on the horizon. I'm up high, and low clouds, fog really, is drifting across. The sun is out, and I'm having another A.T. Moment.

While I've been walking, I've been thinking about some of the A.T. Moments I've had. In particular, the shuttle ride in Erwin, with the Reagge and the purple, cloudy mountains comes to mind. Pure Bliss.

So, what are A.T. Moments?

First, each one is a moment. A tiny parcel of time. I will never again be in this place at this time.

But it's also about a place. A space-time coordinate. And that helps me see that in order to experience an A.T. Moment, you need both the place and the time. It won't work if you are always moving. You need to be in a moment. And you must be in a place. Completely. Not checking email, not browsing off to someplace else, or taking a picture.

Our lives are so conditioned by the constant movement and blurring of both place and time. I think it requires submersion in the real world of moments, and maybe some training, to be able to experience A.T. Moments.

Time to move on to camp before it rains.

Besides time and place, what else goes into A.T. Moments?

The foundation starts with a sense of energy built from the anticipation of the adventure.

And by now, we have developed a mastery of our world, and are confident in it.

Fellow hikers encourage and share with us, and trail angels nourish us in body and mind.

Our pretty extraordinary condition aerobically means are brains are getting a lot more of what they need. The endorphins add to the good feelings. The meditation of the walking clears out our heads.

The sense of freedom we have opens us up to so much.

And then there is the gratitude. To whom or what, I do not know. But I do know we are deeply grateful to be here, now. To experience all of this, here and now.

So, to start off with, we feel pretty darn good.

It is on top of all this that we experience the world. And we experience all of it, not just the narrow slice of what is comfortable. The rain, cold, heat. We are living lives fully and not throwing away the nastier experiences.

Our senses are sharpened. Is this a matter of better blood flow, cleaner air, or training? Probably all of the above.

We become very aware of the land itself. All of its contours and folds. All of its rocks and dirt. And the geological history.

We are surrounded by trees and plants in the "green tunnel", and develop strong connections to them.

We see animals as they study us. We begin to understand their world because it is our world, too. We delight in their existence.

And it is beautiful, so we are attracted to it. Smitten by it all.

So we can now see a lot of the components of

A.T. Moments. But one more thing, and the most important thing. The whole is more than the sum of its parts. That's how I would try to explain the intensity. It's more intense than all of the components summed together.

OK. So that's what I feel. But what does science have to say about all this? A new book, <u>The Nature Fix</u> by Florence Williams does a good job of describing some of the research that reveals incredible things.

Nature is very powerful. Even just looking at nature through a window has profound affects. A study of gallbladder-surgery patients found that some of those who had been assigned to a room with a window view of trees had far better outcomes than those who looked out on a brick wall. The nature viewers needed fewer post-operative days in the hospital, needed less pain medication, and were described in nurses' notes as having better attitudes.

But what is it about looking at nature, even through a window, that is so beneficial? Nature is restful. When we see a natural scene, we relax. It's as if our eyes have an easier time of it. And they do.

Nature reuses everything. So the branching on a tree is similar to the distribution of twigs on a branch, which is similar to the leaves on a twig, and the layout of veins in a leaf. The concept is called fractals. Little trees in there.

Our eyes know this. They have evolved seeing nature for a long time, and they work well with it. In another study, EEG machines were used to watch people's brain waves as they observed patterns. When the patterns most closely matched those in nature, their frontal lobes produced the alpha brain waves of a wakefully relaxed state.

So what happens if, instead of just looking at nature on a screen or through a window, you actually walk around in the woods? Researchers in Japan looked at what happens to our bodies when we take leisurely forrest walks, instead of a similar walk in the city. The forrest walks delivered a 12% decrease in cortisol (stress) levels, a 7% decrease in sympathetic nerve activity ("busy brain"), a 6% decrease in heart rate, and a 1.4% decrease in blood pressure, compared to the city walks.

These were short walks. But one week after I returned from my 4 1/2 month amble, my heart rate was 15% lower, and my blood pressure was

8% lower than when I started. I don't know how much different these readings would have been if I just walked in the city. Actually, it would be kind of tough to find a city walk that would be equivalent.

Nature heals. Our blood contains natural killer immune cells. They send messages to cancer and virus infected cells to die. In a study in Japan, men walked in the woods for 2 hours per day for 3 days. Their NK cells increased 40%! It lasted for 7 days. It was still 15% higher after a month.

I experienced an almost miraculous cure once. I fell and cut my arm. I washed it out, and put a bandaid on it. When I finally took the bandaid off a couple of days later, there was barely a scar. It had been a pretty bad cut. I'm sure it would have taken a couple of weeks to heal at home.

We sure experience a lot of awe on the trial. Awesome thunderstorms, awesome views. Being swallowed up in a landscape like that sure puts you in your small place. But that awe makes you 40% more generous, one study found. Maybe that's why hikers care so much for each other. It's the awe.

But does nature make us smarter? A pilot study

was set up using the Remote Associates Test to measure intuition and creativity. After just 3 days of hiking, participants did 50% better on the test. so maybe that's why people think hikers are so weird. There are some pretty crazy solutions to problems, like socks for mittens.

Science is starting to catch up to what hikers know instinctively. Nature has many benefits. More is better. Most of the long term studies end after one week. That's nothing. After one week, I was just beginning to feel what I would feel after 4 1/2 months. It takes time.

So that's science. What about "beyond science"? In the 1960s, Cleve Backster reported that plants could respond to human thoughts. Though his work was never replicated scientifically, I, for one, believe that communication does happen with people who are tuned into plants. I think that is a lot of what a "green thumb" is. And I have heard stories from people I trust about plants hooked up to garage door openers that respond to their human friend by opening the door on arrival home.

Well, that might be a bit much for you to believe if you have never experienced anything like that. Maybe someday you will.

When I think about A.T. Moments, I would say that almost always, an intense connection was at the heart of it. Those purple, misty mountains near Erwin TN, or the wind blown mists in the Smokies.

And to get all of these benefits, all you have to do is walk.

Caught With My Pants Down

August 7, Waynesboro, VA

Well, I got here a bit earlier than expected. And not in a good way. A bit of negative A.T. Moments.

A few nights ago, we were camping in a beautiful spot near a forest road crossing. Lots of open fields with apple trees, a nice spring, and a place to camp under the pine trees. On the way in, a former thru hiker local guy who was camping nearby gave us a garden tomato to eat, and we sampled the abundant apples, which were ripe. The tomato was incredibly wonderful, so it was a good evening.

But... First, the bugs. Loads of gnats, mosquitos, and even yellow jackets. We missed having our picnic table, and a place to sit, but had a nice dinner, and retired to our tents.

Then, in the middle of the night (full moon, too), when I got up to pee, terrible, explosive diarrhea. Soiled my pants, then cleaned up the best I could, then changed. And then, before morning, soiled my pants again.

Well, anyway, that went on and off for a few days. Had a bit of a reprieve at the Dutch Haus B & B, which was fabulous. But then, a couple of days ago, I ruined my last backup shorts. So it was down to one pair, partially soiled, stinky, and soaking wet from hiking in the rain. And the drinking water was stagnant. Definite negative A.T. Moments.

Then yesterday, when I got to the

north ridge of 3 ridges, I met up
with an eager young day hiker. He
was amazed that we had walked
from GA, and wanted to know
everything about long distance
hiking. He walked with us over to
hanging rock. The view was
mesmerizing, and he was hooked.

We walked to the shelter, where I
was glad to use the privy. He
decided to hike down the Mov-
Haur side trail, a very tough one,
and I decided to eat dinner.

Neither endeavor went well. I
could not finish dinner, and
needed to use the privy again. As
it was getting dark, he was
nowhere to be seen.

Then, just minutes before dark, he
showed up from the opposite
direction. He realized that he did
not have enough time to hike
back, so he hitched back to the

Blue Ridge Parkway, and then hiked back in the 1 1/2 miles.

Well, he did not have a headlamp, and it was getting dark. And I was very frustrated, and wanted to be near some working plumbing. So...

He and I hiked out together using my headlight. He gave me a ride into the inn here. I payed him just what he paid to get back to his car. Net result - I got my ride to plumbing, and he got his rides for free. It worked out perfectly.

So I'm enjoying a vacation from the vacation. Just got back from eating at the Greenleaf. A very nice, sophisticated place with Cab Franc from VA, and Maryland crab cakes and jazz. Definitely looking north now, and it feels good. Hope the antibiotics I got at the clinic (after a 3 hour wait) work quickly so I can head north with Caveman the day after tomorrow, into the Shenandoahs.

It was amazing how quickly the young day hiker we encountered connected with the trail. He was curious, and interested in all of the mechanics of long distance hiking. But once he got to gaze out over Hanging Rock, that was it. Awe does that. It was his first time on the trail, but he was hooked. In that moment, awe. You could see it happen.

When I wrote the journal entry, I was pretty bummed out, so I did not describe the details, which really are quite humorous. Now.

There where only 3 of us in the shelter that morning, me, Caveman, and a section hiker, Old Crow. I had an urgent call of nature, so I marched up the trail to the privy with my roll of toilet paper. Almost got there in time, too.

Well, I was able to do a pretty decent job of cleaning me and the privy up. But those shorts... Forget about it. No way could I put them on again. But I knew my last pair, still wet from hiking in the rain the day before, was hanging on a nail in the shelter.

What to do? I opened the privy door slowly, and looked down the trail to the shelter. Still only Caveman and Old Crow down there. I was not worried about Caveman. We were family by now. But Old Crow?

So I stepped out, and in my best, feral person birthday suit, casually walked down the trail. As I approached the shelter, Old Crow looked up in utter astonishment. Here was this crazy person, stark naked, in front of him. I thought he was going to have a heart attack.

But, with a quick explanation, he understood.

Shit happens on the trail.

Blissful Days

August 16, Rock Spring Cabin,
Shenandoah National Park, VA

I'm sitting at a nice, dry picnic
table, flooded by sun, with a
beautiful view of the Shenandoah
Valley below. The hut is just up
the path from here, and it will be
full tonight. Besides Caveman
and I, there is Just John, the ex-
military man, the young women
from Canada, and Giggles and
Butterscotch. There are also 2
south bounders from Belgium.

It is cool, almost cold, and calm
here. We got rained on getting
here, and the temps have been in
the 70s. So the season is definitely
beginning to change.

And I've been thinking a lot
about home. It seems we are
getting closer now. And in only 2

weeks, I'll see Jose at Lisa's. I sure miss him. I really, really want to be with him and home.

But I want to finish this trail, too. In 2 weeks, we will be at least in Harper's Ferry. What a trip that will be.

Up till today, I really have not been liking Shenandoah National Park very much. Lots of people, shelters full every night, and the sound of motor cycles and cars almost everywhere on skyline drive. And the ridiculous "backcountry" signs. SUVs in backcountry? I don't think so.

But there have been A.T. Moments. Day before yesterday, Gigs, Butterscotch and I lounged at a beautiful overlook at lunch. Felt so good.

And then today, Caveman and I

took the trail out of the Big
Meadows Campground up here. It
is a beautiful trail, built by the
CCC. Stone walls cut into the
cliff. Beautiful! It reminds me of
the Smokies. The trail. The park.
And I remember it took me
awhile to get into that, too. So
hopefully, I'll enjoy it for what it
is. And the black berry shakes
and burgers are great, too!

August 17, in the woods below
Pass Mountain Hut, Shenandoah
National Park

Well, yesterday was a day of
numerous, intense A.T. Moments.

It started with all of us, the
Canadians, Butterscotch, Gigs and
Caveman taking a break on a
beautiful overlook. The day was
dry, cool and clear. Perfect
hiking weather. The view superb.

The company, wonderful.

Then Caveman and I headed up to Stoney Man Overlook. It was a bit busy up there, with some rock climbers getting ready to repel down the cliff. But the view was spectacular!

Then we saw it. A crow was flying - soaring around, noisily squawking at us. Soaring like a hawk.

Then, suddenly, right in front of all those human eyes, she squawked and then flew upside down for a few seconds! Wow, none of us had ever seen that happen before.

Can you imagine the sheer joy of flying - soaring, and then doing a back-flip? I really can't help thinking that she was showing off for us. Look at me! I can fly!

Upside down!

But even if she was not showing off, she sure was enjoying herself on that gorgeous, sunny afternoon that we all enjoyed together.

I'm sure it is a joy to fly. But you know what? It's a joy to walk, too. One foot in front of the other, one step at a time. And you can cross a continent. What a joy!

A beautiful thought on a beautiful day.

Shit Or Get Off the Pot

August 24, Luray, VA

This is a nice town. Friendly people, good restaurants, and the caverns. But I'm ready to get out of here now, and hit the trail. I'm a hiker, after all.

Last Sunday was a tough day. It rained the day before, and the morning dawned in soft drizzle. I needed 4 trips to the privy at night, and one of them came a bit too late. Another cleanup.

So we all stayed in our sleeping bags. Finally, I got the courage to get up, but I did not know what to do. I knew that I did not want this to continue, though. So everyone helped out.

I got the number of a trail angel, Dr. Dick. There was no signal at the Gravel Springs Hut, so I hiked up to Skyline Drive with Caveman. Sure enough, there was a signal up there. Dr. Dick said he could pick me up at the shelter, so I went back down. Around an hour later, he showed up and drove right to the shelter. He checked things out, painted out some graffiti, and drove me here.

I'm hopeful that the stronger antibiotics I'm being treated with will take care of the problem. At least I now know all of the things that my ailment is not.

Tomorrow, Dr. Dick will drive me to the Blackburn Trail Center, where I will rendezvous with Caveman and the Canadians. I can't wait!

August 26, Teahorse Hostel, Harper's Ferry, West Virginia

I've been thinking about this for weeks - months, and now I'm here! I guess that's something.

The hike was not easy. 13.5 miles from Blackburn, with lots of rocks. No climbing, but a large descent, and I'm a bit out of shape.

Last night was fun. Caveman and I had dinner at the Anvil with Smarties and Hatchet, the Canadians, who had by now acquired trail names. I enjoyed being with them so much. It's good to be with my hiking buddies again.

We spent the afternoon down in the historic district, and it was interesting. So much history, architecture, the rivers, the railroad, John Brown. A lot happened here.

On the way back, I had another attack, a very bad one. I sure hope I'm not relapsing. I just can't go on like this. It's time to shit or get off the pot. I decided that if I'm not over this, I'll get out when Lisa picks me up. Just can't go on like this anymore. And I feel terrible thinking this is how it might end. But what else can I do?

Harper's Ferry is almost mythical in hiker lore. It is close to the halfway point, so it is the starting, ending, or midpoint for hikers going either way. The Appalachian Trail Conference is located there, and maintains a register of hikers passing through. They take a photo, which goes into the books they maintain documenting your passage. So Caveman and I are in their book for August 2012. I was proud to have made it there, mostly under my own power.

Somewhere along the way, we met a day hiker we did not like very much. She said that all we were doing was walking. Almost anyone can do that. We did not like her because we knew she was right.

It is true that basically all you have to do is walk. All day. Most of the week. For months. That's all.

Still, it's tough. I think the mental toll is the most costly. You have to have some gumption to keep on truckin, sometimes. And it does get a little... tedious, from time to time.

And it is hard on the body, too. Constant wear and tear. Almost everyone has knee issues at some point. And then there is the starvation.

And, well, the shits. Not uncommon. Lots of poetry and prose about that on the privy walls.

We were mostly eating food we could find in the trail towns. A lot of pasta sides and ramen noodles, embellished any way you could imagine. Have you ever looked at the ingredient list on any of those things? You will need a lot of time to read it, with a chemistry text handy. It does catch up with you eventually. After months.

Have you ever watched a cat or dog shit? How furtive it is. How vulnerable it makes them feel. And for us, too.

So I am grateful for the help I got from Dr. Dick. He would not accept any money for the many miles he drove me. Instead, he suggested I make a donation to PATC (Potomac Appalachian Trail Club), which I did.

And did I mention the starvation?

Well, that is the trail, too.

Last Days

Maryland was a bitter-sweet blur. The walk along the C&O canal was a very different type of trail, and a nice break for us. The view from Weverton Cliffs made Harper's Ferry into a model railroad setup. I'll always remember that 1/2 mile steep climb down to the gusher of a spring at the Ed Garvey Shelter. And we did enjoy the views from the ridge, and the soda machines in the state parks.

But when we got to Ensign Cowall Shelter, the water was stagnant. Since my problem returned, we booked into the nearby Free State Hiker Hostel.

It was a sad day, my last full day on the trail. The next morning, Caveman and I said our goodbyes. He headed north. I headed south, back up to the ridge to say my goodbyes to the trail, after 4 1/2 months.

Ending

September 1, on the ridge south of Ensign Cowall Shelter, Maryland

Well, this is it. The last hour and a half of a 4 and a half month hike. I'm up on the ridge, overlooking the farms below. It's a bucolic quilt of trees, grass, hay and dirt. All is very peaceful here.

I feel like a section hiker again. That is the kind of stuff I always did as a section hiker. Build time in for hours at an overlook. I'm looking forward to that again. I'll get to experience a chunk of the mountains deeply.

But I'm so glad to have done a 4 1/2 month, 1000 mile chunk at once. The flow and connectivity of the A.T. Moments effected me deeply.

Every hike has to end, be it in Maine, CT, NY or Maryland. There will always be a time to fold up the trekking poles.

The view here is peaceful. It could be VT, or more likely, MA, but it is Maryland, the Free State. Fitting place to end my current bondage (and that is what it is!) to this trail. The leaves are already coming off the willow that is growing in the rocks on the ridge (strange place). September is such a nice time to hike.

But September is wonderful at home, too. Make wine. Plant broccoli and fall crops. Get wood.

Time to be home.

And so one of the most significant times of my

life came to a close. Oh sure, I've been on the trail since. And I will be again, over and over. But I'll never be in those same mountains at that same summer of 2012 again.

The path I walked through space-time, over, under, around and through those mountains and days exposed me to more than I could ever put into words, and to feelings I have never felt before. That path is forever etched deeply into the foundation of my being, of who I am. Those months were lived deeply. Emotionally. Intensely. Beautifully. Gratefully.

If you ever feel that life does not seem to have much to offer any more, you have no idea.

All you have to do is walk.

Epilog

After I left the trail, Caveman continued on, all the way to NY state. The Applewoods (#5 and Zen) completed their thru hike in the snow at Harper's Ferry on December 12, 2012. Bee Man completed the entire trail in 2014.

And Will See? I went home and got my internal plumbing working again, and regained the 35 pounds I lost, but it took a year. I continued section hiking in Maine, CT and NY.

And, you ask, when do I expect to finish the trail?

Will see.

All I have to do is walk.

Want to Take a Walk?

Does the story of my hike make you want to go for a hike on the A.T.? As you can see from the map index at the front of the book, the A.T. is close to so many people in the Eastern USA. It might be possible for you to drive to a road crossing, and then do a day hike up to a spectacular view. But be forewarned, you might be captured. By the trail.

A good resource to help you begin your walk, however long it might be, is the Appalachian Trail Conservancy. Their web site, appalachiantrail.org has all kinds of information to help you get started. The ATC is a non-profit organization, and it reflects the spirit of the trail.

The A.T. is a 2,190 miles long national park that goes through 14 states. That is pretty unique, but even more surprising is that it is maintained almost completely by volunteers. There are 31 local trail maintaining clubs that do the work of keeping it open. Maybe that foundation of giving that is so integral to the A.T.'s DNA explains the generosity I experienced on the trail. Or maybe, it is the trail itself that inspires the generosity of all those thousands of people who work so hard for the trail.

But for anyone who has been smitten by the trail, there is a deep, abiding love for it. And it is so precious. We all know we all have to join in and do our part. We need to contribute in any way we can.

This precious resource must be used wisely. The ATC web site has so much practical information about trail use. So please, do consult the web site before you walk, and walk wisely.

Happy Trails!

Acknowledgements

Gratitude. That is a word you have often seen in this book. The trail does that.

This book would not exist without the encouragement of my sister, Lisa Sievel-Otten, who has been urging me to write for as long as I can remember. She also reviewed an early draft, and suggested the title of the book. Diana K. Perkins, a friend and established author, generously gave of her time and advice, and suggested the cover design. Christine Acebo provided transportation to the trail numerous times, as well as the cover photos.

I am very grateful to Bee Man and Indian Brave for their generous work in editing. Caveman's numerous suggestions for additions made this a far better book.

So many helped me during my time on the trail. #5 attended to my minor medical emergencies. Caveman kept me from stepping on rattle snakes, and kept me going with his sense of humor. Dick Hostelley drove me many miles to medical care when I needed it, and returned me back to the trail. I am grateful to all those nameless trail angels that helped me on my journey.

Finally, I will be eternally grateful to my husband, Jose Sobrinho, for his wisdom in understanding my infatuation with the trail, and enduring a four and a half month separation.

www.ingramcontent.com/pod-product-compliance
Lightning Source LLC
Chambersburg PA
CBHW032104280326
41933CB00009B/757